*By the Editors of Consumer Guide®
and Leading Doctors*

The Women's Book of Home Remedies

*With John H. Renner, M.D.,
and the Consumer Health
Information Research
Institute*

PUBLICATIONS INTERNATIONAL, LTD.

CONSULTANT:

John H. Renner, M.D., is the president and medical director of the Consumer Health Information Research Institute (CHIRI), a nonprofit organization dedicated to providing reliable and accurate patient health education for preventive care, wellness, and self-help. Dr. Renner also serves as a member of the Board of Directors of the National Council Against Health Fraud; as clinical professor of family practice at the University of Missouri in Kansas City, Missouri; and as an adjunct professor of preventive medicine at the University of Kansas Medical School in Kansas City, Kansas.

CONTRIBUTING WRITERS:

Sue Berkman is a veteran science/health writer who writes for a variety of consumer and professional publications, including *Woman's Day, Good Housekeeping, Health,* and *Women's Health and Fitness News.* She has also coauthored two books on health.

Linda J. Brown is a freelance writer specializing in health and the environment. She writes an environmental column for *Good Housekeeping,* and her articles have appeared in *Self, Omni,* and other national magazines.

Jenny Hart Danowski researches and writes consumer articles for newsletters and magazines in the areas of health, fitness, and psychology. Her work has appeared in Whittle Communications' health and living publications, *Woman's Day,* and *Men's Health.*

Bobbie Hasselbring is the former editor of *Medical SelfCare* and has authored five books on health and psychology. She currently writes a column for the *Oregonian* and has become a nationally recognized health writer. The American Heart Association awarded her its 1991 Award for Media Excellence.

Susan G. Hauser is a freelance writer who works as a contributing writer to the *Wall Street Journal* and as a special correspondent to *People Magazine.*

Susan Nielsen writes regularly on health and consumer issues for such magazines as *Good Housekeeping* and *Family Circle Magazine.* She has been an associate health editor of *Redbook Magazine,* as well as a senior editor for "The Better Way" section of *Good Housekeeping.*

Brianna L. Politzer is a freelance writer specializing in health, medicine, and nutrition. She has worked as a newspaper reporter and an editor. She has contributed to many health publications, including *Medical Tribune News Service, American Health,* and *AIDS-Patient Care.*

Diana Reese is a medical writer who has written for such national publications as *American Health, Health, Longevity, HealthWatch,* and *Physician's Weekly.* She was previously senior editor on health publications at Whittle Communications.

CONTENTS

MEDICAL AND TECHNICAL ADVISORS

Sabiha Ali, M.D. Neurologist, Houston Headache Clinic, Houston, Texas **David Alpers**, **M.D.** Professor of Medicine and Chief of the Gastroenterology Division, Washington University School of Medicine, St. Louis, Missouri **Peter A. Banks**, **M.D.** Director, Clinical Gastroenterology Service, Brigham and Women's Hospital; Lecturer on Medicine, Harvard Medical School, Boston, Massachusetts **Andrew Baron**, **D.D.S.** Clinical Associate Professor, Lenox Hill Hospital, New York, New York **Evan T. Bell**, **M.D.** Specialist in Infectious Diseases, Lenox Hill Hospital, New York, New York **Richard Bennett**, **M.D.** Assistant Professor of Medicine, Johns Hopkins School of Medicine, Baltimore, Maryland **Wilma Bergfeld**, **M.D.**, **F.A.C.P.** Head, Clinical Research, Department of Dermatology, Cleveland Clinic Foundation, Cleveland, Ohio **Henry J. Bienert**, **Jr.**, **M.D.** Orthopedic Surgeon, Tulane University School of Medicine, New Orleans, Louisiana **Henry Blackburn**, **M.D.** Mayo Professor of Public Health and Professor of Medicine, University of Minnesota, Minneapolis, Minnesota **Richard C. Bozian**, **M.D.** Director of Research, Monarch Foundation, Cincinnati, Ohio; Professor of Medicine, Assistant Professor of Biochemistry, Director, Division of Nutrition, University of Cincinnati, Cincinnati, Ohio **Earl J. Brewer**, **Jr.**, **M.D.** Former Head, Rheumatology Division, Texas Children's Hospital, Houston, Texas; Former Clinical Professor, Former Head, Rheumatology Division, Department of Pediatrics, Baylor College of Medicine; Author, *Parenting a Child with Arthritis* **Vera Brown** Skin-Care Expert; Author, *Vera Brown's Natural Beauty Book* **W. Virgil Brown**, **M.D.** Past President, American Heart Association; Professor of Medicine, Director, Division of Arteriosclerosis and Lipid Metabolism, Emory University School of Medicine, Atlanta, Georgia **John Buse**, **M.D.**, **Ph.D.** Assistant Professor, Department of Medicine, Section of Endocrinology, University of Chicago; Director, Endocrinology Clinic, University of Chicago Medical Center, Chicago, Illinois **C. Wayne Callaway**, **M.D.** Member, 1989–1990 Dietary Guidelines Advisory Committee to the U.S. Department of Agriculture/Department of Health and Human Resources; Associate Clinical Professor of Medicine, George Washington University, Washington, D.C. **David B. Carmichael**, **M.D.** Medical Director, Cardiovascular Institute, Scripps Memorial Hospital, La Jolla, California **William P. Castelli**, **M.D.** Director,

Framingham Heart Study, Framingham, Massachusetts **Michael Castleman** Former Editor, *Medical SelfCare* magazine; Author, *Cold Cures* **Col. Ernest Charlesworth, M.D.** Assistant Chief of Allergy and Immunology, Wilford Hall U.S. Air Force Medical Center, San Antonio, Texas **Daniel S.J. Choy, M.D.** Assistant Clinical Professor of Medicine, Columbia University College of Physicians and Surgeons; Director, Laser Laboratory, St. Luke's–Roosevelt Hospital Center, New York, New York **Amanda Clark, M.D.** Assistant Professor of Obstetrics and Gynecology, Oregon Health Sciences University, Portland, Oregon **Jack W. Clinton, D.M.D.** Associate Dean of Patient Services, Oregon Health Sciences University School of Dentistry, Portland, Oregon **Peter F. Cohn, M.D.** Chief of Cardiology, State University of New York at Stony Brook Health Sciences Center, Stony Brook, New York **Cheryl Coleman, R.N., B.S.N., I.C.C.E.** Director, Public Relations, International Childbirth Education Association; Childbirth Educator, Hillcrest Medical Center, Tulsa, Oklahoma **Sonja Connor, M.S., R.D.** Coauthor, *The New American Diet*; Research Associate Professor, School of Medicine, Oregon Health Sciences University, Portland, Oregon **Paul Contorer, M.D.** Chief of Dermatology, Kaiser Permanente; Clinical Professor of Dermatology, Oregon Health Sciences University, Portland, Oregon **James R. Couch, Jr., M.D., Ph.D.** Professor and Chairman, Department of Neurology, University of Oklahoma Health Sciences Center, Oklahoma City, Oklahoma **Donald R. Coustan, M.D.** Professor and Chair, Obstetrics and Gynecology, Brown University School of Medicine; Chief, Obstetrics and Gynecology, Women and Infants Hospital of Rhode Island, Providence, Rhode Island **Jeffrey A. Cutler, M.D.** Hypertension Specialist and Chief, Prevention and Demonstration Research Branch, National Heart, Lung, and Blood Institute, National Institutes of Health, Bethesda, Maryland **Joseph C. D'Amico, D.P.M.** Podiatrist, New York, New York **John Staige Davis IV, M.D.** Margaret Trolinger Professor of Medicine, University of Virginia School of Medicine, Charlottesville, Virginia **Barbara Deskins, Ph.D, R.D.** Associate Professor of Clinical Dietetics and Nutrition, University of Pittsburgh, Pittsburgh, Pennsylvania **Seymour Diamond, M.D.** Founder, Diamond Headache Clinic, Chicago, Illinois **Alan M. Dietzek, M.D.** Vascular Surgeon, North Shore University Hospital, Manhasset, New York; Assistant Professor of Surgery, Cornell Medical College, New York, New York **Cornelius P. Dooley, M.D.** Gastroenterologist, Santa Fe, New Mexico **Roland C. Duell, D.D.S., M.S.** Professor of Endodontics, Department of Oral Health Practice, University of Kentucky College of Dentistry, Lexington, Kentucky **Harry S. Dweck, M.D.** Director, Regional Neonatal Intensive Care Unit, Westchester Medical Center; Professor of Pediatrics, Associate Professor of Obstetrics and Gynecology, New York Medical College, Valhalla, New York **Johanna Dwyer, D.Sc., R.D.** Director, Frances Stern Nutrition Center, New England

Medical Center Hospitals; Professor, Tufts University School of Nutrition; Professor, Tufts University Medical School, Boston, Massachusetts **Rose Dygart** Cosmetologist; Barber; Hair-Care Instructor; Manicurist; Owner, Le Rose Salon of Beauty, Lake Oswego, Oregon **Victor G. Ettinger, M.D.** Medical Director, Bone Diagnostic Centres, Torrance and Long Beach, California **Alexander A. Fisher, M.D., F.A.A.D.** Author, *Contact Dermatitis*; Clinical Professor of Dermatology, New York University Medical Center, New York, New York **Rosemarie L. Fisher, M.D.** Professor of Medicine, Division of Digestive Diseases, Yale University School of Medicine, New Haven, Connecticut **Steven C. Fiske, M.D.** Past President, New Jersey Gastroenterological Society; Associate Professor of Medicine/Gastroenterology, Seton Hall University School of Postgraduate Medicine; Assistant Clinical Professor of Medicine and Gastroenterology, University of Medicine and Dentistry of New Jersey, Newark, New Jersey **Sharon Fleming, Ph.D.** Associate Professor of Food Science, Department of Nutritional Sciences, University of California at Berkeley, Berkeley, California **Raven Fox, R.N., I.B.C.L.C.** Registered Nurse and Lactation Consultant, Evergreen Hospital Medical Center, Kirkland, Washington **Phyllis Frey, A.R.N.P.** Nurse Practitioner, Bellevue, Washington **Lawrence S. Friedman, M.D.** Associate Professor of Medicine, Jefferson Medical College, Thomas Jefferson University, Philadelphia, Pennsylvania **Clifton T. Furukawa, M.D.** Past Chairman, Professional Education Council, American Academy of Allergy and Immunology; Clinical Professor of Pediatrics, University of Washington School of Medicine, Seattle, Washington **Glenn B. Gastwirth, D.P.M.** Deputy Executive Director, American Podiatric Medical Association, Bethesda, Maryland **Hugh Gelabert, M.D.** Assistant Professor of Surgery, Section of Vascular Surgery, University of California at Los Angeles School of Medicine, Los Angeles, California **Ruby Ghadially, M.D.** Assistant Clinical Professor, Department of Dermatology, University of California at San Francisco, San Francisco, California **David N. Gilbert, M.D.** Director, Chiles Research Institute; Director, Department of Medical Education, Providence Medical Center, Portland, Oregon **Donald Girard, M.D.** Head, Division of General Internal Medicine, Oregon Health Sciences University, Portland, Oregon **W. Paul Glezen, M.D.** Pediatrician, Influenza Research Center, Professor of Microbiology and Immunology, Professor of Pediatrics, Chief Epidemiologist, Baylor College of Medicine, Houston, Texas **Billy Glisan, M.S.** Director, Injury Prevention Program, Texas Back Institute, Dallas, Texas **Alan H. Gluskin, D.D.S.** Associate Professor and Chairperson, Department of Endodontics, University of the Pacific School of Dentistry, San Francisco, California **Arthur I. Grayzel, M.D.** Senior Vice-President for Medical Affairs, Arthritis Foundation, Atlanta, Georgia **Sadja Greenwood, M.D.** Assistant Clinical Professor, Department of Obstetrics, Gynecology, and Reproductive

Sciences, University of California at San Francisco, San Francisco, California **Sandra Hazard, D.M.D.** Managing Dentist, Willamette Dental Group, Inc., Oregon **Robert P. Heaney, M.D.** John A. Creighton University Professor, Creighton University, Omaha, Nebraska **James A. Hearn, M.D.** Assistant Professor of Medicine, University of Alabama at Birmingham, Birmingham, Alabama **Mindy Hermann, R.D.** Spokesperson for the American Dietetic Association **Sherman Hess, B.S., R.Ph.** Registered Pharmacist and Manager, Hillsdale Pharmacy, Portland, Oregon **Rose Hust** Osteoporosis Coordinator, Knoxville Orthopedic Clinic, Knoxville, Tennessee **Pascal James Imperato, M.D.** Professor and Chairman, Department of Preventive Medicine and Community Health, State University of New York Health Science Center, Brooklyn, New York **Janna Jacobs, P.T., C.H.T.** President, Section on Hand Rehabilitation, American Physical Therapy Association (APTA) **Katherine Jeter, Ed.D., E.T.** Executive Director, Help for Incontinent People (HIP), Union, South Carolina **Conrad Johnston, M.D.** Chief, Division of Endocrinology and Metabolism, Indiana University School of Medicine, Indianapolis, Indiana **Stephen R. Jones, M.D.** Chief of Medicine, Good Samaritan Hospital and Medical Center; Associate Professor of Medicine, Oregon Health Sciences University, Portland, Oregon **Marcia Kielhofner, M.D.** Clinical Assistant Professor of Medicine, Baylor College of Medicine, Houston, Texas **Albert M. Kligman, M.D., Ph.D.**

Emeritus Professor of Dermatology, University of Pennsylvania School of Medicine, Philadelphia, Pennsylvania **Matthew J. Kluger, Ph.D.** Professor of Physiology, University of Michigan Medical School, Ann Arbor, Michigan **Albert B. Knapp, M.D., F.A.C.P.** Adjunct Assistant Attending Physician, Lenox Hill Hospital, New York, New York; Instructor in Medicine, New York Medical College, Valhalla, New York **Kermit E. Krantz, M.D.** University Distinguished Professor, Professor of Gynecology and Obstetrics, Professor of Anatomy, University of Kansas Medical Center, Kansas City, Kansas **Jerold Lancourt, M.D.** Orthopedic Surgeon, North Dallas Orthopedics & Rehabilitation, P.A., Dallas, Texas **Ira J. Laufer, M.D.** Clinical Associate Professor of Medicine, New York University School of Medicine; Medical Director, The New York Eye and Ear Infirmary Diabetes Treatment Center, New York, New York **Paul Lazar, M.D.** Professor of Clinical Dermatology, Northwestern University School of Medicine, Chicago, Illinois **Harold E. Lebovitz, M.D.** Professor of Medicine, Chief of Endocrinology and Diabetes, Director, Clinical Research Center, State University of New York Health Science Center, Brooklyn, New York **Theodore Lehman, M.D.** Associate Clinical Professor of Surgery (Urology), Oregon Health Sciences University; Director, The Oregon Impotence Center, Portland, Oregon **Suzanne M. Levine, D.P.M.** Podiatrist, New York, New York **Jerome Z. Litt, M.D.** Author, *Your Skin: From Acne to Zits*; Assistant Clinical

Professor of Dermatology, Case Western Reserve University School of Medicine, Cleveland, Ohio **Gabe Mirkin, M.D.** Author, "The Mirkin Report," a monthly newsletter on health, fitness, and nutrition; Associate Professor, Georgetown University Medical School, Washington, D.C. **Anthony Montanaro, M.D.** Associate Professor of Medicine, Division of Allergy and Immunology, Oregon Health Sciences University, Portland, Oregon **Alan N. Moshell, M.D.** Director, Skin Disease Program, National Institute of Arthritis and Musculoskeletal and Skin Diseases, National Institutes of Health, Bethesda, Maryland **Willibald Nagler, M.D.** Anne and Jerome Fisher Physiatrist-in-Chief, Chairman of the Department of Rehabilitation Medicine, The New York Hospital–Cornell Medical Center, New York, New York **Luis Navarro, M.D.** Author, *No More Varicose Veins*; Founder and Director, Vein Treatment Center, New York, New York **Harold Neu, M.D.** Professor of Medicine and Pharmacology, Columbia University College of Physicians and Surgeons, New York, New York **Noreen Heer Nicol, M.S., R.N., F.N.C.** Senior Clinical Instructor, University of Colorado Health Sciences Center School of Nursing; Dermatology Clinical Specialist/Nurse Practitioner, National Jewish Center for Immunology and Respiratory Medicine, Denver, Colorado **Nelson Lee Novick, M.D.** Author, *Super Skin: A Leading Dermatologist's Guide to the Latest Breakthroughs in Skin Care*; Associate Clinical Professor of Dermatology, Mount Sinai School of Medicine, New York, New York

Edward J. O'Connell, M.D. Past President, American College of Allergy and Immunology; Professor of Pediatrics, Allergy/Immunology, Mayo Clinic, Rochester, Minnesota **Richard Ottaviano** President, Covermark Cosmetics, Moonachie, New Jersey **Mary Papadopoulos, D.P.M.** Podiatrist, Alexandria, Virginia **Frank Parker, M.D.** Professor and Chairman, Department of Dermatology, Oregon Health Sciences University, Portland, Oregon **Nalin M. Patel, M.D.** Author of *The Doctor's Guide to Your Digestive System*; Clinical Instructor, University of Illinois at Urbana–Champaign, Champaign, Illinois **Robert A. Phillips, M.D., Ph.D.** Director, Hypertension Section, Associate Director, Cardiovascular Training Program, Division of Cardiology, Mount Sinai Medical Center, New York, New York **Neville R. Pimstone, M.D.** Chief of Hepatology, Division of Gastroenterology, University of California Davis, Davis, California **Deborah Purcell, M.D.** Past Chair, Department of Pediatrics, St. Vincent Hospital and Medical Center, Portland, Oregon **Gayle Randall, M.D.** Assistant Professor of Medicine, Department of Medicine, University of California, Los Angeles, School of Medicine, Los Angeles, California **Basil M. Rifkind, M.D., F.C.R.P.** Chief, Lipid Metabolism and Atherogenesis Branch, National Heart, Lung and Blood Institute, National Institutes of Health, Bethesda, Maryland **Margaret Robertson, M.D.** Staff Physician, St. Vincent Hospital and Medical Center, Portland, Oregon **Norton Rosensweig, M.D.** Associate

Clinical Professor of Medicine, Columbia University College of Physicians and Surgeons, New York, New York **Peter K. Sand, M.D.** Associate Professor of Obstetrics and Gynecology, Northwestern University School of Medicine; Director, Evanston Continence Center, Evanston Hospital, Evanston, Illinois **Marvin Schuster, M.D.** Professor of Medicine with Joint Appointment in Psychiatry, Johns Hopkins University School of Medicine; Chief, Division of Digestive Diseases, Francis Scott Key Medical Center, Baltimore, Maryland **James Shaw, M.D.** Chief, Division of Dermatology, Good Samaritan Hospital and Medical Center; Associate Clinical Professor of Medicine, Oregon Health Sciences University, Portland, Oregon **Fred D. Sheftell, M.D.** Director and Founder, The New England Center for Headache, Stamford, Connecticut **Elyse Sosin, R.D.** Supervisor of Clinical Nutrition, Mount Sinai Medical Center, New York, New York **Thomas J. Stahl, M.D.** Assistant Professor of General Surgery, Georgetown University Medical Center, Washington, D.C. **Felicia Stewart, M.D.** Coauthor, *My Body, My Health* and *Understanding Your Body*; Gynecologist, Sacramento, California **David M. Taylor, M.D** Author, *Gut Reactions: How to Handle Stress and Your Stomach*; Assistant Professor of Medicine, Emory University, Atlanta, Georgia; Assistant Professor of Medicine, Medical College of Georgia, Augusta, Georgia **Joseph Tenca, D.D.S., M.A.** Past President, American Association of Endodontists; Professor and Chairman, Department of Endodontics, Tufts University School of Dental Medicine, Boston, Massachusetts **Abba I. Terr, M.D.** Clinical Professor of Medicine, Director, Allergy Clinic, Stanford University Medical Center, Stanford, California **Frank J. Veith, M.D.** Professor of Surgery, Chief, Vascular Surgical Services, Montefiore Medical Center–Albert Einstein College of Medicine, New York, New York **Ken Waddell, D.M.D.** Dentist, Tigard, Oregon **Douglas C. Walta, M.D.** Gastroenterologist, Portland, Oregon **John R. Ward, M.D.** Professor of Medicine, University of Utah School of Medicine, Salt Lake City, Utah **Kimra Warren, R.D.** Outpatient Dietitian, St. Vincent Hospital and Medical Center, Portland, Oregon **Miles M. Weinberger, M.D.** Director, Pediatric Allergy and Pulmonary Division, University of Iowa Hospitals and Clinics, Iowa City, Iowa **Thelma Wells, Ph.D., R.N., F.A.A.N., F.R.C.N.** Professor of Nursing, University of Rochester School of Nursing, Rochester, New York **Ted Williams, M.D.** Media spokesperson, American Academy of Pediatrics; Pediatrician, Dothan, Alabama **Ronald Wismer, D.M.D.** Past President, Washington County Dental Society; Dentist, Beaverton, Oregon **Susan Woodruff, B.S.N.** Childbirth and Parenting Education Coordinator, Tuality Community Hospital, Hillsboro, Oregon **Harold Zimmer, M.D.** Obstetrician and Gynecologist, Bellevue, Washington **Jane Zukin** Author, *The Dairy-Free Cookbook* and *The Newsletter for People with Lactose Intolerance and Milk Allergies*

FOREWORD

The Women's Book of Home Remedies is a valuable health advisory manual. It is holistic, in the correct sense of the word—it offers preventive medicine tips as well as sound nutrition, medical, mental, dental, cosmetic, and stress-reduction advice.

The home remedies that are described in this book are not "miracle" cures or risky alternative therapies done over your doctor's objections, nor are they meant to take the place of the advice and treatments prescribed by your health-care providers. Rather, they are safe, practical actions that you can take to help yourself with your own health care. They are designed to help you prevent, cope with, and/or treat 40 common health problems. They can save you money on health-care costs. They can help to keep you healthy, wealthy, and wise.

How much this book helps you, however, depends on how you use it. As you read and use this book and as you take more responsibility for your own health care, keep the following important points in mind:

• Remember that there are no doctor "secrets" in this book. All of the physicians and health-care providers openly and easily shared their recommendations without payment or promise. Discuss these ideas with your own doctor to see if he or she thinks these are valid for you. Use this book to improve communication with your health-care providers. This book is loaded with practical ideas. Your doctor will be interested in your use of them.

• Be careful of "self" diagnosis. Work with your doctor on your diagnosis. Even a doctor has a "fool for a patient" if he treats himself.

• Don't try every remedy listed for your condition on every condition you have. Especially, don't put everything listed for your skin on your skin—you could end up with a new medication rash. Go slowly; use common sense.

• Heed the warnings included with the remedies. These warnings are carefully written to help you avoid harm or quackery. Pay special attention to the boxes labeled "Hello, Doctor?" These include special warnings and can help alert you to conditions and symptoms that require a doctor's attention.

The Women's Book of Home Remedies has been carefully compiled. It contains information currently held to be true and helpful. As medicine and scientific experience grow, we may learn to do some things differently. Learn along with us. Continue to practice good, safe, self-help techniques based on scientific opinions and facts. Continue to maintain an open dialogue with your health-care providers. Continue to read, to ask questions, and to be an active, informed participant in your own health care.

John H. Renner, M.D.
President
Consumer Health Information Research Institute
Kansas City, Missouri

ALLERGIES

28 Ways to Feel Better

Spring's pollens. Summer's smog. Autumn's falling leaves. Winter's house dust. For millions of Americans, each change of season brings its own brand of allergens and irritants. For people with common hay fever and allergies, these pollutants can bring on symptoms ranging from a continuous, annoying postnasal drip to a full-scale, coughing-sneezing-itchy-eyed allergy attack. For other allergy sufferers, such as those with allergic asthma or an allergy to bee stings, attacks can be fatal.

In many cases, allergy symptoms are difficult to differentiate from the symptoms of other disorders and illnesses, such as a cold, a deformity of the nose, or a food intolerance. For this reason, many doctors suggest that allergies be properly diagnosed by a board-certified allergist (a medical doctor who treats allergies) to avoid the self-administration of inappropriate medications or other remedies. Also, many allergy sufferers can benefit from today's wide range of available treatments, such as new prescription antihistamines that don't cause drowsiness, nasal corticosteroids, and allergy injections that can provide immunity to a specific allergen (an allergen is the name for any substance, such as pollen, that causes an allergic reaction). If you don't go to the doctor, you may be missing out on a treatment that may be of great help to you.

However, many mild allergies, such as seasonal hay fever or an allergy to cats, can be treated with a combination of properly used, over-the-counter antihistamines and a wide range of strategies to reduce or eliminate your exposure to particularly annoying allergens.

The following tips are designed to help reduce the discomfort caused by the most common allergies. They may be used in combination with an allergist's treatment or, if your allergies are mild, by themselves.

Avoid the culprit. Sometimes, the best way to reduce the discomfort of an allergy is to avoid exposure to the allergen as much as possible, according to Edward J. O'Connell, M.D., professor of pediatrics at the Mayo Clinic in Rochester, Minnesota, and past president of the

HELLO, DOCTOR?

If your allergies are causing you to cough, wheeze, and have trouble breathing, you should see an allergist, says Abba I. Terr, M.D., a clinical professor of medicine and director of the Allergy Clinic at Stanford University Medical Center in California. "You may have allergic asthma, which really has to be supervised by a doctor," he says. People with allergic asthma, which is sometimes mistaken for bronchitis, must often be prescribed inhalers and other drugs. Trying to self-treat may be dangerous, Terr says.

American College of Allergy and Immunology. "Take all practical measures," he says. For example, if you are allergic to cats, avoid visiting the homes of friends who own them. If you must be around a cat, make the visit as short as possible and avoid touching or picking up the animal, he says.

Rinse your eyes. If your eyes are itchy and irritated and you have no access to allergy medicine, rinsing your eyes with cool, clean water may help soothe them, O'Connell says. Although not as effective as an antihistamine, this remedy certainly can't do any damage.

Try a warm washcloth. If sinus passages feel congested and painful, a washcloth soaked in warm water may make things flow a little easier, according to O'Connell. Place the washcloth over the nose and upper-cheek area and relax for a few minutes, he suggests.

Use saline solution. Irrigating the nose with saline solution may help soothe upper-respiratory allergies by removing irritants that become lodged in the nose, causing inflammation, according to Anthony Montanaro, M.D., associate professor of medicine in the Division of Allergy and Immunology at Oregon Health Sciences University in Portland. "The solution may also remove some of the inflammatory cells themselves," he adds.

Wash your hair. If you've spent long hours outdoors during the pollen season, wash your hair after you come inside to remove pollen, suggests Clifton T. Furukawa, M.D., clinical professor of pediatrics at the University of

Washington School of Medicine in Seattle and past chairman of the Professional Education Council for the American Academy of Allergy and Immunology. The sticky stuff tends to collect on the hair, making it more likely to fall into your eyes.

Take a shower. If you wake up in the middle of the night with a coughing, sneezing allergy attack, a hot shower may wash off any pollen residues you've collected on your body throughout the day, says Furukawa. The warm water will also relax you and help you go back to sleep, he adds.

Wear sunglasses. On a windy day in pollen season, a pair of sunglasses may help shield your eyes from airborne allergens, according to O'Connell. For extra protection, try a pair of sunglasses with side shields or even a pair of goggles.

Beware of the air. "Air pollution may augment allergies and may actually induce people to have allergies," Montanaro says. He recommends staying outside as little as possible on smoggy days or wearing a surgical mask, especially if you exercise outside. "The mask won't remove everything, but it will help," he adds.

Make your house a no-smoking zone. "Don't allow smoking in your house or apartment," O'Connell says. Tobacco smoke is a notorious irritant, either causing or aggravating respiratory allergies.

Keep the windows shut. Most Americans, except for those who have jobs that keep them outdoors, spend most of their time inside. During pollen season, this can be a terrific advantage for those with pollen allergies, according to O'Connell. "The bottom line, for pollen allergies, is keeping the windows shut," he says. "Closed windows will keep pollen out of the house or apartment. For pollen sufferers, during the pollen season, there is really no such thing as fresh air." Air purifiers may help eliminate indoor pollen, but they tend to stir up dust, he adds.

Filter your vacuum. "It is very important to not recycle the allergy factors back into your home as you clean," says Furukawa. "For example, you're not doing much good

BUST THE DUST

The following tips from Edward J. O'Connell, M.D., can help you rid your bedroom of dust mites—microscopic insects that live in dusty, humid environments. The feces and corpses of the mites are thought to be the irritating components in dust. Allergists believe that since we spend most of our time at home in the bedroom, that's the most important place to allergy-proof.

Encase pillows and mattresses. Invest in airtight, plastic or vinyl cases or special covers that are impermeable to allergens for your pillows and mattresses (except for waterbeds). Pillows and mattresses contain fibrous material that is an ideal environment for dust-mite growth. These cases are usually available at your local department store or through mail-order companies. You can also contact the Asthma and Allergy Foundation of America for more information on where to purchase cases and covers.

Wash your bedding. Down, kapok, and feather comforters and pillows are out for people with allergies. The feathers have a tendency to leak and can wreak havoc with your respiratory tract. Comforters and sheets should be washed every seven to ten days in as hot water as they'll tolerate. Wash your mattress pads and synthetic blankets every two weeks.

Clean once a week. Putting off cleaning for longer than this may allow an excessive amount of dust to collect. However, since cleaning raises dust, it's best not to clean more than once a week. If necessary, spot dust with a damp cloth more often.

Avoid overstuffed furniture. "If the bedroom's decor lends itself to it, add more wood and vinyl furniture and avoid over-stuffed furniture," O'Connell says. Since carpeting makes an excellent dust-mite lair, opt instead for bare floors or ask your doctor about a prescription product for killing mites in carpets.

Choose washable curtains. If possible, invest in curtains that can be washed, since dust mites often hide in their fabric.

Vacuum the venetians. The slats of venetian blinds are noto-rious dust collectors. If you can't replace your venetian blinds with washable curtains, at least run the vacuum lightly over them or dust them well during your thorough weekly cleaning.

Don't use the bedroom as storage space. Stored items tend to collect dust. If the bedroom is the only storage space you have, wrap items tightly in plastic garbage bags.

Clean out your air conditioner and heating ducts. Every month or so, clean out the vents on your heating and air-condi-tioning units, or have someone clean them for you. These ducts are breeding grounds for mold, dust mites, and bacteria.

if your vacuum cleaner allows small particles of dust to be blown back into the air as you vacuum." He recommends putting a filter on the exhaust port of your vacuum, if your machine is the canister type (uprights don't usually have an exhaust port). If dust really bothers you and you've got the money, you can invest in an industrial-strength vacuuming system, Furukawa says. Some allergists recommend a brand called Nilfisk, he adds, which has an excellent filtering system and retails for about $500. To find out where you can purchase filters or special vacuums, talk to your allergist or write to the Asthma and Allergy Foundation of America, Department CG, 1125 15th Street NW, Suite 502, Washington, D.C., 20005.

Dust with a damp cloth. Dusting at least once a week is important—but if done improperly, it may aggravate respiratory allergies, O'Connell says. He recommends avoiding the use of feather dusters, which tend to spread dust around, and opting instead to contain the dust with a damp cloth. Dusting sprays may give off odors that can worsen allergies, he adds.

IS IT A FOOD ALLERGY?

Do you feel congested after you eat dairy products? Does red meat make you feel sluggish? Does sugar give you a headache? If you answered "yes" to any of these questions, you probably don't have a food allergy.

"There's a big difference between what the public perceives as a food allergy and what is really a food allergy," says Anthony Montanaro, M.D. "The distinction is important, since a real food allergy can kill you and a food intolerance can't."

If you are truly allergic to a food, the reaction will be almost immediate, occurring from within a few minutes to two hours after you eat it, according to Abba I. Terr, M.D. The most common symptoms, he says, are hives, diffuse swelling around the eyes and mouth, or abdominal cramps. A less common symptom is difficulty breathing. In severe cases, extremely low blood pressure, dizziness, or loss of consciousness may result. In these instances, a call for an ambulance or other emergency medical assistance is warranted.

Don't dust at all. If dusting aggravates your allergies, don't do it. Instead, ask a spouse or family member to do the dirty work, or hire a housekeeper, if possible, O'Connell recommends.

Dehumidify. "Dust mites (microscopic insects that are usually the allergy culprits in dust) grow very well in humid areas," O'Connell says. He recommends investing in a dehumidifier or using the air conditioner, which works equally well. A dehumidifier can also help prevent mold, another allergen, from growing. When cooking or showering, take advantage of the exhaust fan—another way to help keep humidity to a minimum.

Think before you burn. Although it is common to burn household and construction refuse, this may not be such a wise idea, says Furukawa. "Wood that is treated with heavy metals or other chemical-laden materials will irritate everybody, but the person who is allergic or asthmatic will have proportionately more difficulty," he says. "Also, pay attention to what you are throwing in the fireplace." Of course, your best bet is to stay away from the fireplace when it's in use.

Cut through the smoke. Many people with respiratory allergies find that wood smoke poses a particular problem, Furukawa says. With wood stoves, the biggest problem is "choking down" the stove, or decreasing the amount of oxygen in order to cool down the fire, he explains. Choking down throws irritating toxins into the air, which will be breathed in by you and your neighbors.

Leave the lawn mowing to someone else. During pollen season, a grass-allergic person is better off letting someone else—anyone else—mow the lawn, Montanaro says. "Find out when the pollination season in your area is," he advises. "Here in the Northwest, I tell people not to mow between May and the Fourth of July."

Wash your pet. A little-known trick for cat or dog owners who are allergic to fur: Bathe your pet frequently. "There is strong evidence that simply bathing the animal in warm water substantially reduces the amount of allergen on the animal's fur," Furukawa says. "Animals se-

CHOOSING AND USING AN OVER-THE-COUNTER ANTIHISTAMINE

If you've got your doctor's OK to use them, over-the-counter antihistamines can be an economical way to relieve your allergy misery. However, many people misuse these drugs, believing them to be an on-the-spot fix for whenever they feel itchy-eyed or sneezy.

"The problem with antihistamines is, most people wait until they're miserable, then take one and don't find they work," says Miles M. Weinberger, M.D., director of the Pediatric Allergy and Pulmonary Division at the University of Iowa Hospitals and Clinics in Iowa City. "If you have classical ragweed hay fever, you'll get the maximum benefit from antihistamines if you start taking them a week or two before the allergy season begins." (The timing of the allergy season depends on where you live; consult your doctor about when the allergy season occurs in your part of the country.)

As for what type of antihistamine to use, Weinberger recommends chlorpheniramine maleate, which is found in many over-the-counter preparations (check the list of ingredients on the package). Chlorpheniramine maleate is one of the oldest, safest allergy drugs with a proven track record, he says. It can take care of symptoms such as sneezing; itchy, runny nose; and itchy eyes. (If you also have nasal stuffiness, says Weinberger, you might try a combination product that contains chlorpheniramine and pseudoephedrine, a nasal decongestant.) He suggests starting with a dose of perhaps one-fourth of what the package recommends, then slowly building up to 24 milligrams per day (12 milligrams in the morning and 12 milligrams in the evening), providing you can maintain that dosage without drowsiness. Since drowsiness tends to go away in a week or two, Weinberger recommends starting with evening doses, then adding a morning dose as you begin to tolerate the medication. (Be sure to avoid operating a motor vehicle or heavy machinery if you find that the medication makes you drowsy.) "Approximately 75 percent of the people with pollen symptoms will get quite adequate relief with a 24 milligram dosage," Weinberger says.

Edward J. O'Connell, M.D., agrees that antihistamines work best when they are used as preventive medicine. For people with pet allergies who know they will be exposed to someone else's cat or dog, he recommends taking antihistamines beginning 10 to 14 days in advance.

crete substances from their sweat glands and their saliva—it is water soluble and you can rinse it off." If you're a cat owner and can't imagine bathing your beloved feline for fear of being scratched near to death, take heart: Furukawa says that in an informal survey that he conducted, he discovered that one out of ten cats will purr when bathed. If they are started as kittens, chances are higher that bath time will be a harmonious experience, he says. He recommends a bath in warm water, with no soap, once every other week.

In addition to bathing your pet, try to wash your hands soon after you've had direct contact with your furry friend.

Make sure your final rinse really rinses. Chemicals in detergents and other laundry products can cause skin irritation in many people, O'Connell says. "There really are no mild detergents," he explains. "It's important that the final rinse cycle on your machine thoroughly rinses the detergent from your clothes."

Call ahead. When planning a vacation or business trip, call ahead to find a room that will be easier on your allergies. Ask for a room that's not on the lower level, because a room on the lower level may have been flooded in the past and may still be a haven for mold growth. Shop around for a hotel or motel that doesn't allow pets, so you won't be subject to the leftover dander of the last traveler's dog or cat. If possible, bring your own vinyl- or plastic-encased pillow.

ARTHRITIS

44 Coping Strategies

An estimated 37 million Americans are caught in the grip of some form of arthritis or rheumatic disease. And few of us will make it to a ripe old age without joining the fold. If one of these diseases has a hold on you, read on. While there are no cures, there are steps you can take to ease discomfort and get back more control over your life. There are more than 100 different forms of arthritis and rheumatic disease, with a host of causes, according to the Arthritis Foundation in Atlanta. Among the more widely known afflictions are osteoarthritis, rheumatoid arthritis, gout, and lupus.

Osteoarthritis is primarily marked by a breakdown and loss of joint cartilage. Cartilage is the tough tissue that separates and cushions the bones in a joint. As cartilage is worn away and the bones begin to rub against each other, the joint becomes aggravated. In osteoarthritis, this breakdown of cartilage is accompanied by minimal inflammation, hardening of the bone beneath the cartilage, and bone spurs (growths) around the joints. "It will eventually affect virtually everyone in old age," says John Staige Davis IV, M.D., professor in the Division of Rheumatology at the University of Virginia School of Medicine in Charlottesville.

Rheumatoid arthritis, on the other hand, is not an inevitable aspect of the aging process. For reasons unknown, the synovial membrane, or lining, of a joint becomes inflamed, so pain, swelling, heat, and redness occur.

In gout, needle-shaped uric acid crystals collect in the joints, due to a fault in the body's ability to process purines. Purines are naturally occurring chemicals found in certain foods, such as liver, kidney, and anchovies. The disease primarily affects overweight, fairly inactive men over age 35.

Lupus, on the other hand, affects many more women than men. It is a condition in which the body's own immune system attacks healthy cells. The symptoms are wide-ranging, from joint pain to mouth sores to persistent fatigue.

Researchers are beginning to understand what may predispose some people to arthritis. One clue to the puzzle: "There are indications that collagen, which helps form the body's cartilage, may be defective in some people," says Arthur I. Grayzel, M.D., senior vice-president for Medical Affairs at the Arthritis Foundation.

While you can't cure your condition, you can adopt coping techniques that will leave you more active and in control.

EASING STIFFNESS AND DISCOMFORT

Here are some tips to help relieve discomfort and get you back into the swing of things.

Keep moving. Maintain movement in your joints as best you can. This can help keep your joints functioning better for a longer amount of time and, at the same time, brighten your outlook on life. "Every patient should keep active," says John R. Ward, M.D., professor of medicine at the University of Utah School of Medicine in Salt Lake City. "And remember that even small movements mean a lot. If all you can tolerate is a little housecleaning or gardening, for instance, that's OK, too."

Exercise, exercise, exercise. "Exercises work best when inflammation has calmed down," notes Janna Jacobs, P.T., C.H.T., physical therapist, certified hand therapist, and president of the Section on Hand Rehabilitation of the American Physical Therapy Association (APTA).

There are a few different types of exercises that are used to help arthritis sufferers. The simplest, easiest exercises that can be done by almost any arthritis sufferer are called range-of-motion exercises. They help maintain good movement by putting the joints through their full range of motion. You'll find several range-of-motion exercises recommended by the Arthritis Foundation in "Exercises for Arthritis" on page 24.

Isometrics, in which you create resistance by tightening a muscle without moving the joint, can help to strengthen muscles. Weight-bearing exercises, such as walking, also build muscle strength. While strengthening exercises can be beneficial for the arthritis sufferer, however, they should only be done under the supervision and care of a therapist or physician, says Grayzel. And, "anyone with any type of cardiovascular disease should not do multiple resistance exercises for a sustained amount of time," warns Ward.

Stretching, which helps make the muscles more flexible, is often recommended as the first step in any exercise regimen. Likewise, warming up your joints before beginning any exercise makes them more flexible. Massage your muscles and/or apply hot or cold compresses or both—whichever your health-care practitioner recommends or you prefer. Or try a warm shower. (See "Heat or Cold: Which Is Best?" on page 26.)

EXERCISES FOR ARTHRITIS

These exercises are recommended by the Arthritis Foundation. For best results, carry out the exercises in a smooth, steady, slow-paced manner; don't bounce, jerk, or strain. Don't hold your breath; breathe as naturally as possible. Do each exercise five to ten times, if possible. If any exercise causes chest pain, other pain, or shortness of breath, stop. When your joints are inflamed, it's best to skip the exercises and rest. If you have any questions, contact your therapist or physician. And remember: It may be some time before you feel the benefits of regular exercise, so be patient with yourself.

Shoulders: Lie on your back and raise one arm over your head, keeping your elbow straight. Keep your arm close to your ear. Return your arm slowly to your side. Repeat with the other arm.

Knees and hips: Lie on your back with one knee bent and the other as straight as possible. Bend the knee of the straight leg and bring it toward the chest. Extend (straighten) that same leg into the air and then lower it to the floor. Repeat with the other leg.

Hips: Lie on your back with your legs straight and about six inches apart. Point your toes up. Slide one leg out to the side and return, keeping your toes pointing up. Repeat with the other leg.

Knees: Sit on a chair that's high enough so you can swing your legs. Keep your thigh on the chair and straighten out your knee. Hold a few seconds. Then bend your knee back as far as possible to return to the starting position. Repeat with the other knee.

Ankles: Sit on a chair and lift your toes off the floor as high as possible while keeping your heels on the floor. Then return your toes to the floor and lift your heels as high as possible. Repeat.

Fingers: Open your hand with your fingers straight. Bend all the finger joints except the knuckles. Touch the top of the palm with the tips of your fingers. Open and repeat.

Thumbs: Open your hand with your fingers straight. Reach your thumb across your palm until it touches the base of the little finger. Stretch your thumb out again and repeat.

Give your hands a water workout. Try doing your hand exercises in a sink full of warm water for added ease and comfort, suggests Jacobs.

Don't overdo it. Ward has come up with a "useful recipe" you can use to see if you've overdone your exercise routine. See how you feel a few hours after you exercise and then again after 24 hours. If your pain has increased considerably during that period of time, then it's time to cut back on the frequency and amount of exercise that you're doing, he says. Of course, if the activity brought relief, you've found a worthwhile exercise. Tailor your routine to include the exercises that give you the most relief—and the most enjoyment.

Play in a pool. If you find that even simple movements are difficult for you, a heated pool or whirlpool may be the perfect environment for exercise (unless you also have high blood pressure, in which case you should avoid whirlpools and hot tubs). Try a few of your simpler exercises while you are in the water. The buoyancy will help reduce the strain on your joints. And, "the warm water will help loosen joints and maintain motion and strength," says Ward. Even a warm bath may allow you some increased movement. In a pinch, a hot shower may do: Running the stream of water down your back, for instance, may help to relieve back pain.

Don't overuse over-the-counter creams. These nonprescription pain-relieving rubs give temporary relief by heating up the joints. However, "frequent use may activate enzymes that can break down the cartilage in the joints," says Davis.

Put on a scarf. Not around your neck, but around the elbow or knee joint when it aches. "A wool scarf is your best bet," says Jacobs. Be careful not to wrap it too tightly, however; you don't want to hamper your circulation.

Pull on a pair of stretch gloves. "The tightness caused by the stretchy kind may, in fact, reduce the swelling that often accompanies arthritis," says Ward. And the warmth created by covered hands may make the joints feel better. "Wearing thermal underwear may have the same warming effect on joints," says Grayzel.

Get electric gloves. Hunters use these battery-operated mitts to keep their hands toasty on cold mornings in the woods. "The gloves just may do the trick to keep your hands warm and pain-free," says Jacobs. She recommends keeping them on all night while you sleep.

HEAT OR COLD: WHICH IS BEST?

There are no hard and fast rules when it comes to deciding which—heat, cold, or a combination of the two—will give you the best results. The bottom line, says John R. Ward, M.D.: "Do whichever feels the best." Here are some guidelines that may help you decide.

Heat relieves pain primarily by relaxing muscles and joints and decreasing stiffness. In some instances, however, heat may aggravate a joint that's already "hot" from inflammation, as is sometimes the case with rheumatoid arthritis. On the other hand, osteoarthritis causes minimal inflammation and may respond well to heat application. If you find that your compress cools down too quickly, you may want to try methods that offer more consistent heating. An electric blanket or heating pad, for example, can provide sustained dry heat. A warm shower, bath, or whirlpool can keep the wet heat coming. And using some method of warmth to loosen up the muscles before exercise can help them perform better.

Cold treatment is ordinarily used to reduce pain in specific joints. Cold application should not be used with vasculitis (inflammation of the blood vessels) or Raynaud's phenomenon (a condition, characterized by spasms of the arteries in the fingers and toes, that may occur in conjunction with rheumatoid arthritis) without a doctor's approval, however. There are many ways to make a cold pack: You can fill a plastic bag with crushed ice, use a package of frozen peas or frozen unpopped popcorn, or use a package of blue ice, for example. Apply the cold pack, wrapped in a thin towel, to only one or two joints at a time, so that you don't get a chill.

You may find that alternating heat and cold gives you the most relief. For the best results, the Arthritis Foundation recommends the contrast bath: Soak your hands and feet in warm water (no more than 110 degrees Fahrenheit) for about three minutes, then soak them in cold water (about 65 degrees Fahrenheit) for about a minute. Repeat this process three times, and finish with a warm-water soak.

Try a water bed. According to the National Water Bed Retailers' Association in Chicago, many owners claimed in a study that their rheumatoid arthritis "was helped very much by a water bed." And Earl J. Brewer, Jr., M.D., former head of the Rheumatology Division of Texas

Children's Hospital in Houston, believes he knows why. "The slight motions made by a water bed can help reduce morning stiffness," he says. "And a heated water bed may warm the joints and relieve joint pain."

Slip into a sleeping bag. If a water bed is out of the question, you might consider camping gear. "The cocoonlike effect of a sleeping bag traps heat, which can help relieve morning aches and pains," reports Brewer. He learned of its therapeutic effects when many of his patients told him that they got relief by sleeping in their sleeping bags on top of their beds.

Get "down." Brewer tells the story of a doctor from Norway who happened to stay in a bed-and-breakfast while on business in New York. The doctor, who was suffering from arthritis pain, slept peacefully each night in the B&B's bed and woke each morning pain-free. The bed was outfitted with a goose-down comforter and pillow. According to Brewer, the bedding's warmth and minute motion brought on the relief. For those who are allergic to down, an electric blanket may bring some relief.

Watch your weight. Being overweight puts more stress on the joints. As a matter of fact, a weight gain of 10 pounds can mean an equivalent stress increase of 40 pounds on the knees. So if you are carrying excess pounds, losing weight can help improve joint function. "People who lose weight can slow the progress of their osteoarthritis," says Grayzel.

Question any cure-all. Frustrated by the chronic pain of arthritis, some sufferers pursue a litany of promises for 100 percent relief—whether from a so-called miracle drug, a newfangled diet, or another alternative treatment. Unfortunately, at this time, arthritis has no cure. So, before you jump at the next hot-sounding testimonial, proceed with caution. Get all the facts. Consult your physician or other health-care provider. Even age-old techniques, such as wearing a copper bracelet, should be viewed with skepticism, agree most experts. And remember, if something sounds too good to be true, it probably is.

PROTECTING YOUR JOINTS

In addition to easing discomfort, you can learn to live well with arthritis by protecting your joints. What's more, with a little planning and reorganizing, you can learn to do daily tasks more efficiently, so that you'll have more energy to spend on activities you enjoy. Here are some tips from the Arthritis Foundation that can help.

Plan ahead each day. Prepare a realistic, written schedule of what you would like to accomplish each day. That way, you can carry out your most demanding tasks and activities when you think you'll have the most energy and enthusiasm—in the morning, for instance.

Spread the strain. As a general rule, you want to avoid activities that involve a tight grip or that put too much pressure on your fingers. Use the palms of both hands to lift and hold cups, plates, pots, and pans, rather than gripping them with your fingers or with only one hand. Place your hand flat against a sponge or rag instead of squeezing it with your fingers. Avoid holding a package or pocketbook by clasping the handle with your fingers. Instead, grasp your goods in the crook of your arm—the way a football player holds the ball as he's running across the field—and you won't be tackled by as much pain.

Avoid holding one position for a long time. Keeping joints "locked" in the same position for any length of time will only add to your pain and stiffness. Relax and stretch your joints as often as possible.

"Arm" yourself. Whenever possible, use your arm instead of your hand to carry out an activity. For example, push open a heavy door with the side of your arm rather than with your hand and outstretched arm.

Take a load off. Sitting down to complete a task will keep your energy level up much longer than if you stand.

Replace doorknobs and round faucet handles with long handles. They require a looser, less stressful grip to operate, so you'll put less strain on your joints.

Build up the handles on your tools. For a more comfortable grip, tape a layer or two of thin foam rubber, or a foam-rubber hair curler, around the handles of tools.

Choose lighter tools. Lightweight eating and cooking utensils can keep your hands from getting heavy with hurt.

Let automatic appliances do the work for you. Electric can openers and knives, for instance, are easier to operate than manual versions. An electric toothbrush has a wider handle than a regular toothbrush.

Say no to scrubbing. Spray pots and pans with nonstick cooking spray and/or use cookware with a nonstick surface. Consider getting a dishwasher, too, to save your joints some work.

Keep your stuff within easy reach. Adjust the shelves and racks in any storage area so that you don't have to strain to reach the items you need. Buy clothes with pockets to hold things you use often and need close by, like a pair of glasses. Use an apron with pockets to carry rags and lightweight cleaning supplies with you as you do your household chores. Store cleaning supplies in the area in which they will be used. Keep the same supplies in several places, such as the upstairs bathroom and the downstairs bathroom as well as the kitchen.

Use a "helping hand" to extend your reach. For those items you can't store nearby, buy a long-handled gripper, the kind used in grocery stores to grab items from top shelves. Make household chores easier with a long-handled feather duster or scrub brush. Grab your clothes from the dryer with an extended-reach tool.

Don't overdo the housework. Plan on tackling only one major cleaning chore a day, whether it is doing the laundry or cleaning the kitchen.

Velcro is the way to go. Interlocking cloth closures on clothing and shoes can save you the frustration of buttoning and lacing.

Walk this way up and down the stairs. Lead with your stronger leg going up, and lead with your weaker leg coming down.

Bend with your knees. When reaching for or lifting something that's low or on the ground, bend your knees and keep your back straight as you lift.

Let loose with loops. You won't need to use quite as tight a grip if you put loops around door handles, such as those on the refrigerator and the oven. Have loops sewn on your socks, too, then use a long-handled hook to help you pull them up.

Dig out that little red wagon. Heavier loads will be out of your hands if you use a wagon or cart that glides along on wheels. Use it to tote groceries or baskets of laundry, for instance.

Read with ease. Lay your newspaper out on the table rather than holding it up to read. Likewise, lay a book flat or use a book stand to give your hands a break as you read.

Sit on a stool in the tub. A specially made stool can give you a steady place to shower and can ease your way in and out of the tub.

Plant yourself on a stool in the garden. Sitting, rather than stooping, over your flower beds or vegetable garden may help reduce the stress on your back and legs.

Ask for help. Don't be afraid to ask your family members or friends for assistance when you need it. As the saying goes, many hands make light work. By sharing the load, you'll have more time and energy for the people and activities you enjoy.

Contact the Arthritis Foundation. The Arthritis Foundation can let you know of joint-friendly or energy-saving items specially made for use by arthritis sufferers. Call the Arthritis Foundation Information Line at 800-283-7800, Monday through Friday, 9:00 A.M. to 7:00 P.M. Eastern time, to talk to a skilled operator who can answer your questions about arthritis.

BACK PAIN

19 Ways to Keep Back Pain at Bay

Maybe you lifted something heavy or swung a golf club a little too enthusiastically. Or maybe you've been sitting in an uncomfortable desk chair for two weeks, sweating over a deadline. Whatever the reason, now you're flat on your back, wishing for something—anything—that will put an end to the agony.

Take heart—you're not alone. Almost every American suffers from back pain at some point in his or her life. The bad news is that unless you have a major injury or disc problem, your doctor may not be able to do much for you other than prescribe some pain medication and advise you to rest. The good news is that by following some simple steps, you can be on your feet again in just a few days. Even better, you can avoid having to endure similar discomfort in the future.

EASING THE PAIN

The following remedies are appropriate for anyone who is suffering from back pain as a result of tight, aching muscles or a strain. However, if you are experiencing pain, weakness, or numbness in the legs or a loss of bowel or bladder control, see a doctor without delay.

Go to bed. "Bed rest is a way of removing the strain from the muscles," says Daniel S. J. Choy, M.D., director of the Laser Laboratory at St. Luke's–Roosevelt Hospital Center and an assistant clinical professor of medicine at Columbia University College of Physicians and Surgeons in New York. "The back muscles' job is to hold you erect. If you lie down, it takes the stress off of the muscles." The best way to lie is flat on your back with two pillows underneath your knees. Never lie facedown, Choy says, since this position forces you to twist your head to breathe and may cause neck pain. Make an effort to get up and start moving around after three days, since longer periods of bed rest may make the muscles weaker and more prone to strain, he adds.

Ice it. Applying an ice pack to the painful area within 24 hours of the injury can help keep inflammation and discomfort to a minimum, according to Willibald Nagler, M.D., Anne and Jerome Fisher Physiatrist-in-Chief and chairman of the Department of Rehabilitation Medicine at The New York Hospital–Cornell Medical Center in New York. "Ice does one thing—it decreases the nerve's ability to conduct a painful stimulus," he says. Nagler suggests wrapping ice cubes in a plastic bag, then applying the bag on top of a thin towel that has been placed on the skin. Leave the ice pack on for 20 minutes, take it off for 30 minutes, then replace it for another 20 minutes.

Take a hot bath. If more than 24 hours have passed since the injury occurred, ice will not help reduce pain or inflammation. After that time, heat may help increase the elasticity of the muscles by about ten percent, Nagler says. Jerold Lancourt, M.D., an orthopedic surgeon at North Dallas Orthopedics & Rehabilitation, P.A., in Dallas, tells his patients to soak in a hot bath for 20 minutes or more. Pregnant women, however, should not sit in a hot bath for too long, since raising the body temperature over 100 degrees Fahrenheit for long periods may cause birth defects or miscarriage.

Invest in a new mattress. A soft, sagging mattress may contribute to the development of back problems or worsen an existing problem, according to Henry J. Bienert, Jr., M.D., an orthopedic surgeon at Tulane University School of Medicine in New Orleans. If a new mattress is not in your budget, however, a three-quarter-inch-thick piece of plywood placed between the mattress and box spring may help somewhat. "The verdict's not back yet on water beds," he adds. In any case, try to sleep on your back with two pillows underneath your knees.

Get a massage. If you're lucky enough to have an accommodating spouse, friend, or roommate, ask him or her to give you a rubdown. "Lie facedown and have someone knead the muscles," Choy says. Local massage therapists may also make house calls. You can check the yellow pages for listings or ask a friend for a referral.

Relax. Much back pain is the result of muscles made tight by emotional tension, Lancourt says. He recommends that his patients practice relaxation and deep-breathing exercises, such as closing their eyes, breathing deeply, and counting backward from 100.

Take two aspirin. Taking an over-the-counter analgesic such as aspirin, acetaminophen, or ibuprofen may help relieve your pain. However, be aware that not all medications—not even nonprescription ones—are for everyone. Pregnant women, for example, should not take any medication without first checking with their doctor. And people with ulcers should stay away from analgesics containing aspirin, according to Lancourt. "Any medicine should be taken with knowledge of its side effects," he says. "Make sure to get the advice of your doctor."

PREVENTING FUTURE PAIN

Many of the activities you engage in each day—sitting, lifting, bending, carrying—can put a strain on your back. By learning new ways of going about these activities, you can help prevent back pain and ensure the health of your back for years to come. The tips that follow can help.

Use a cushion. "The seats of most cars and trucks are not well designed," Choy says. "They should support the small of your back." If your seat doesn't, Choy suggests that you buy a small cushion that can be fitted to provide the missing support. He adds that the most desirable sitting position is not one in which your back is straight up and down. It's better to be leaning back at an angle of about 110 degrees. If you sit for long hours, Choy also recommends that you periodically get up and walk around.

Put your arm behind your back. If you have to sit for long periods in a chair that doesn't support your lower back and you don't have a cushion, try rolling up a towel or sweater so that it has about the same circumference as your forearm. Then slide the rolled-up cloth between your lower back and the chair, recommends Billy Glisan, M.S., an exercise physiologist and the director of injury prevention programs for the Texas Back Institute in Dallas. In a pinch, you can simply slide your forearm between your lower back and the back of the chair to ease the strain on your back. Even with the best back support, however, sitting is still stressful on your back, so try to make small adjustments in the curvature of your lower back every few minutes or so, advises Glisan.

Swim. Swimming is the best aerobic exercise for a bad back, according to Choy. Doing laps in the pool can help tone and tighten the muscles of the back and abdomen.

BACK-SAVING EXERCISES

The following back exercises were provided by exercise physiologist Billy Glisan, M.S. For best results, do the exercises daily, and don't discontinue them, even after the pain gets better, since strength and flexibility can only be maintained through consistent exercise. Stretches may be done twice a day. Although these exercises are safe and effective for most back pain caused by muscle strain or spasm, Glisan cautions that people with disc or other structural problems should not engage in any type of exercise without advice from their doctor.

Single Knee-to-Chest: Lie on your back with your knees bent and your feet on the floor. Grasp the back of one thigh with both hands; gently and slowly pull toward your chest until you feel mild tension—not to the point of pain. Hold to the count of ten, without bouncing, then release. Repeat four to five times with the same leg, then switch sides. This exercise is a good warm-up to the other exercises.

Double Knee-to-Chest: Lie on your back with your knees bent and your feet on the floor. This time, grasp both thighs, and gently and slowly pull them as close to your chest as you can. Again—pull only to the point of slight tension, and don't bounce. Hold to the count of ten, then release. Repeat four or five times before proceeding to the next exercise.

Lumbar Rotation: Lie on your back with your hips and knees bent, your feet flat on the floor, and your heels touching your buttocks. Keeping your knees together and your shoulders on the floor, slowly allow your knees to rotate to the right, until you reach a point of mild tension. Hold for a count of ten, then return to the starting position. Repeat four to five times on the right side, then switch to the left.

Partial Sit-Up: Lie on your back with your knees bent, your feet flat on the floor, and your hands gently supporting your head. Slowly curl up just to the point where your shoulders come off the floor. Avoid bending your neck. Hold for a few counts, then roll slowly back down. Remember to breathe as you do the exercise. Repeat 10 to 15 times.

Active Back Extension: Lie on your chest on the floor. You can put a pillow under your stomach (not under your hips) if that feels comfortable. Put your arms at your sides, with your hands next to your buttocks. Slowly extend your head and neck and raise your upper body slowly off the floor. Hold for five to ten counts. Slowly lower yourself back to the starting position. Breathe as you do the exercise. Repeat five to ten times.

Walking is second best, he says. You can also try the "Back-Saving Exercises."

Lift with your knees bent. The large muscles of your legs and buttocks are better equipped to bear heavy weights than your back muscles are, according to Bienert. "Pretend you have a goldfish bowl filled with water on the top of your head," he says. "When you squat down to pick something up, don't spill a drop." Bienert also recommends strengthening leg and buttock muscles to facilitate squatting.

Carry objects close to your body. When picking up and carrying heavy objects, pull in your elbows and hold the object close to your body, Choy recommends. "If you have to reach something on a shelf, get right under it and rest it on your head," he says. "Then, the weight is carried by the erect spine, and you don't ask as much of your muscles."

Stay alert. Careless activity is the number-one cause of back injury, according to Lancourt. "If you have had previous back pain, be very careful," he says. "Avoid bending and twisting and lifting. Avoid being caught off guard. Sometimes it's better to hire somebody to do things, such as yard work or carrying heavy suitcases, than to hurt yourself and miss three months of work."

Watch your weight. Maintaining your ideal weight may help take the strain off the back muscles, according to Bienert. "The less you have to carry, the less load you have," he says. "Secondly, when you gain weight in your abdomen, you may become sway-backed, which can accentuate back pain."

BLADDER INFECTION

15 Self-Care Techniques

You have to go, and you have to go *now*. Come to think of it, it seems like you've had to go every 15 minutes since you woke up this morning. And each time, it's been the same story. Not much comes out, but it burns like crazy. What in the world is going on?

If you have pain or burning on urination, the frequent urge to urinate, and/or blood in your urine, chances are you have a bladder infection (also called cystitis, urinary tract infection, or UTI). These symptoms may also be accompanied by lower abdominal pain, fever and chills, and an all-over ill feeling.

Bladder infections are caused by a bacterial invasion of the bladder and urinary tract. "The urine in the bladder is normally sterile," explains Amanda Clark, M.D., assistant professor of obstetrics and gynecology at Oregon Health Sciences University in Portland. "However, if it becomes contaminated with bacteria, a bladder infection can develop."

If you're a woman who suffers from bladder infections, you're not alone. "Women tend to suffer more bladder infections than men because the female urethra, the tube leading from the bladder to the outside of the body, is only about one-and-a-half inches long—a short distance for bacteria to travel," says Sadja Greenwood, M.D., a women's health specialist and assistant clinical professor in the Department of Obstetrics, Gynecology, and Reproductive Sciences at the University of California at San Francisco. (A man's urethra is about eight inches long.) Frequently, the urinary tract becomes contaminated with *Escherichia coli,* bacteria that are normally present in the bowel and anal area. In 10 to 15 percent of cases, bladder infections are caused by another organism, such as *Chlamydia trachomatis.*

Women also suffer more bladder infections because sexual intercourse can irritate the urethra and contribute to the transport of bacteria from the anal area and vagina into the bladder. "We don't really know exactly why intercourse increases the risk of bladder infections," says Clark. "We think it might make the bladder tissues a little more receptive to having an infection or it may cause more bacteria to move up the urethra."

Women who use the diaphragm for birth control have a greater risk of bladder infections, too, says Clark. The diaphragm presses against the neck of the bladder, which inhibits normal urination, she says. As urine flow decreases, pressure within the bladder increases, and the bladder is unable to completely empty itself. The pooled urine then acts as a growth medium for bacteria.

Pregnant women are also more likely to suffer from bladder infections. The changing hormones of pregnancy and the pressure exerted by the enlarged uterus on the bladder and ureters (the two tubes that carry urine from the kidneys to the bladder) put pregnant women at greater risk.

Men can also suffer from this malady. In men, bladder infections are almost always secondary to an infection of the prostate gland (prostatitis), according to Theodore Lehman, M.D., a urologist in private practice and director of The Oregon Impotence Center in Portland. "Primary infection of the bladder in men just doesn't happen, because the bladder is well protected," explains Lehman. "But the prostate sits right in front of the bladder, and bacteria can get into it—through sexual intercourse, trauma like bouncing on a bicycle seat, or some kind of blockage—and it stirs up an infection in the prostate. Then the prostate infection can 'move upstream,' if you will, and infect the bladder."

In men, prostate infection usually feels like "you're sitting on a brick," says Lehman. When the infection extends to the bladder, the symptoms of irritation, urinary frequency, and pain and burning on urination join the achy-bottom feeling.

Bladder infections can often be treated at home with the self-care tips that follow. However, if your symptoms persist for more than 24 hours, if they don't respond to home remedies, or if you suspect that your symptoms may be due to a sexually transmitted disease or other infection, be sure to see your physician.

Load up on fluids. At the first sign of bladder infection, start drinking water and don't stop. During the first 24 hours, Greenwood recommends drinking at least one eight-ounce glass of water every hour. People who suffer from recurrent bladder infections usually don't drink enough liquids. So even when you don't have an active infection, you should make a habit of drinking eight tall glasses of water every day.

According to Lehman, drinking lots of fluid not only dilutes the urine, giving bacteria less to feed on, it also has a "washout" effect on bacteria. "The more bacteria you can wash out," says Lehman, "the less there will be to reproduce."

HELLO, DOCTOR?

In many cases, bladder infections can be successfully treated at home with the remedies described here. However, call your doctor if you:

- Have a personal history of kidney disease
- Are diabetic
- Are pregnant or may be pregnant
- Have shaking spells or have vomited within the last 12 hours (may indicate kidney infection or septicemia, a bacterial infection in the blood that can be fatal)
- Have symptoms and fever that increase after 48 hours of home treatment
- Have blood in your urine
- Have had an abdominal or back injury within two weeks prior to the onset of your symptoms (may indicate kidney injury)
- Have high blood pressure
- Are male and over age 50
- Have or suspect that you have a sexually transmitted disease

Clark warns, however, that people who suffer from urinary leakage (incontinence) probably shouldn't increase their fluids. She says it can make the bladder infection and the incontinence worse.

Have a cranberry cocktail. If you've never developed a taste for the sweet tanginess of cranberry juice, now's the time. Cranberry juice (without added sugar) may make urine more acidic and less hospitable for bacterial growth, says Clark. Drinking cranberry juice is also a way to increase your fluid intake.

Go, go, go. Lehman advises both men and women to avoid what he calls "L.A.-freeway-driver bladder." "Many people don't urinate when they first get the urge because it's inconvenient or there isn't the time or place," he says. "Take a guy who gets off work, has a couple of cups of coffee or a couple of beers, and gets on the freeway in rush-hour traffic. He feels the urge to urinate, but he can't get off the freeway. When he finally gets home and urinates, it's difficult and it burns. By the next day, he's calling his doctor with a prostate infection."

Holding urine allows it to concentrate in the bladder, creating a perfect medium for bacterial growth. In older men, holding urine can cause congestion, inflammation, and obstruction of the prostate and can eventually lead to a prostate infection or sometimes a bladder infection.

Not urinating at the first urge also causes the bladder to distend and stretch. "Essentially, the bladder is a hollow muscle," says Lehman. "If you repeatedly stretch it, then it won't void completely and creates a place for bacteria to grow."

Heat it up. For lower abdominal pain, use a heating pad or hot-water bottle or take a hot bath, advises Greenwood. Lehman says that heat not only relieves the symptoms, it also brings more blood with white blood cells and other infection-fighting blood products to the affected area. (Pregnant women, however, should not sit in a hot bath or hot tub for too long, since raising the body temperature above 100 degrees Fahrenheit for long periods may cause birth defects or miscarriage.)

Take a bath. If you have a lot of burning, a warm "sitz" bath (sitting in three to four inches of water) can ease the pain.

Take a break. Rest in bed, especially if you have a fever. You'll conserve energy and speed healing.

Wear cotton underwear. Cotton underwear, cotton-lined panty hose, and loose clothing will allow the genital area to breathe and stay dry. For men, boxer-type shorts rather than jockey-style shorts are better if prostate and bladder infections are a problem.

Avoid alcohol. Alcohol is a urinary tract irritant for both men and women and should be avoided during a bladder infection.

What about spicy foods, tea, and coffee? Clark says, "They really shouldn't hurt a bladder infection." However, the caffeine in coffee, tea, and colas does stimulate the kidneys to produce more urine and makes the bladder fill up faster during a time when urination is painful. If caffeine seems to make your symptoms worse, avoid it until the infection goes away.

Take a pain reliever. Bladder infections can be painful. Acetaminophen, ibuprofen, or aspirin, especially if taken at bedtime, can ease the pain.

Wash up, lovers. Both partners should wash up before intercourse.

Urinate after lovemaking. If you suffer from recurrent bladder infections, urinate immediately before and after intercourse, advises Clark. This can help flush out bacteria that may have entered the urinary tract.

Switch birth-control methods. Women who use a diaphragm and suffer from recurrent infections should try switching to condoms or a cervical cap. "If you have recurrent bladder infections, see your doctor to have your diaphragm's fit rechecked," says Clark. "You may do better with a smaller diaphragm or a cervical cap."

Keep a bladder-infection diary. If you suffer from recurrent bladder infections, keep a diary to discover what patterns precede an attack. Some people find that their infections are related to stress, menstruation, lovemaking, or other factors. Once you discover what precipitates your infections, you can make changes to alter those patterns.

Wipe from front to back. Most women wipe from back to front, which moves bacteria from the rectum dangerously close to the urethra.

Use condoms. Prostate infection, which can lead to bladder infection, is more common among men with multiple sex partners. Practice safe sex, and always use condoms with partners.

BLISTERS

18 Ways to Treat—and Beat—Them

You just couldn't resist a bargain. Those shoes looked great with your new outfit, even if they didn't feel so great on your feet. "They'll stretch out," you told yourself, and then patted yourself on the back for getting such a good deal.

Unfortunately, you got more than you bargained for—namely, painful blisters to go with your new shoes.

Blisters are tender spots that fill up with fluid released by tiny blood vessels in an area where delicate skin tissues have been burned, pinched, or just plain irritated. Virtually everyone has experienced friction blisters, the kind caused by hot, sweaty, or ill-fitting shoes. If you have one now, read on to find out how to take care of it. Then continue reading to learn how you can help protect your tender tootsies in the future.

TREATING YOUR BLISTER

A blister is your body's way of telling you that skin and tissues are being injured. So while you take steps to relieve the discomfort, you also need to protect the injured area.

Make a tent. Instead of simply placing an adhesive bandage right on top of the blister, "tent" the bandage by bringing in its sides so the padding in the middle of the bandage raises up a bit. "This will not only protect the blister but allow air to circulate, which will aid in healing," says Nelson Lee Novick, M.D., associate clinical professor of dermatology at the Mount Sinai School of Medicine in New York.

Use a double-duty bandage. Another type of bandage, available in pharmacies, contains a gel and antiseptic to cushion and "clean" the blister, says Wilma Bergfeld, M.D., head of clinical research in the Department of Dermatology at the Cleveland Clinic Foundation in Ohio. Ask your pharmacist about it.

Let it breathe. Some physicians believe that a blister should not be covered at all for maximum aeration. Jerome Z. Litt, M.D., assistant clinical professor of dermatology at Case Western Reserve University School of Medicine in Cleveland, is one such doctor. He even suggests slipping your shoe off while you sit at your desk at work in order to give your blister some air.

Smear on ointment. Whether you cover your blister or not, apply an antibacterial/antibiotic ointment to it. Doctors generally recommend Bacitracin or Polysporin, which may be less likely to cause an allergic reaction or sensitivity than other over-the-counter ointments.

BLISTERS

Pad it. When a blister is in an annoying spot, like the bottom of the foot, padding might provide more of a cushion than just a bandage would, advises Bergfeld. She suggests using the circular pads of foam adhesive found in the foot-care aisle of drugstores. "Pharmacies also carry sheets of padding that you can cut to size for a more exact fit," says Bergfeld. Cut the padding in the shape of a donut, and place it on the skin surrounding the blister so the blister fits in the hole. Then gently cover the blister with an antibacterial ointment and bandage.

Put it up. Elevating the blistered area can help relieve the pressure, advises Bergfeld.

Be patient. Expect it to take about a week to ten days for the blister's fluid to be reabsorbed by the body.

Drain it. While some doctors believe that a blister should never be popped because of the risk of infection, most agree that a blister causing extreme pressure—such as one on a toe—is a candidate for draining.

If you should decide to pop it, first wipe the blister and a sewing needle with alcohol. "Never sterilize a needle over a flame," says Novick. "It can create soot on the tip of the needle, which can 'tattoo,' or dirty, the blister." Prick the blister once or twice near its edging; then slowly and gently press out the fluid.

Keep the roof on it. Once you have popped the blister and drained the fluid, do not remove the deflated top skin. This skin, called the blister's roof, protects the blister from infection and forms a "bridge" for new cells to migrate across on their journey to heal the site.

Soak first. To drain a blister on a tough-skinned area, such as the sole of the foot, Litt suggests first soaking the blister in Burow's solution, available from pharmacies in packets or tablets (follow the directions on the package). He recommends soaking the blister for 15 minutes, three to four times a day. A day or two of this will soften the blister and make draining easier.

Watch for signs of infection. Redness, red streaks, or pus in an intact or a "popped" blister should be treated by a doctor.

PREVENTING BLISTERS

Here are ways to prevent friction blisters, according to Glenn B. Gastwirth, D.P.M., Deputy Executive Director of the American Podiatric Medical Association in Bethesda, Maryland:

Buy shoes in the afternoon. "Over the course of the day, your feet may swell by as much as half a shoe size," says Gastwirth. When trying on shoes, wear the same type of socks that you plan to use with the shoes.

Look for leather. Unlike nonporous vinyl and plastic materials, leather has microscopic pores that allow air to circulate, keeping the foot drier. In the same way, so do the clusters of perforated holes primarily found on many styles of sports footwear. A dry foot is less likely to develop blisters.

Don't exercise at midday. The heat of midday, especially in the summer, can make the feet perspire more, making them more blister-prone.

Never wear wet shoes. The wetness can cause more "dragging" between the foot and shoe and can result in blisters. If you jog twice a day, for instance, you may want to buy a second pair of running shoes to wear on your second run each day.

Protect "hot spots." If you have a chronic "hot spot," or place where blisters tend to develop, apply petroleum jelly to it, then slip on your sock. Foam or felt pads, used alone, can also absorb the friction and protect a hot spot. For best results, make sure the padding covers more area than you think a blister would take up, since the neighboring areas can become irritated, too.

Wear the right socks. Specially made sport socks with extra padding in hot spots can help prevent blisters. Natural fibers such as cotton and wool tend to keep the feet dry by absorbing moisture. However, according to Gastwirth, recent research suggests that acrylic fibers may, through a wicking action, actually move moisture away from the foot, keeping it drier and making it less prone to blistering. Your best bet? Try a pair of each and see which type of fiber keeps your feet drier and more comfortable. In addition, make sure the sock fits your foot, so there is less chance of it bunching up inside the shoe and causing a blister.

Try a sprinkle. Foot powders may aid in keeping the foot dry and preventing painful blisters from forming.

BREAST DISCOMFORT
6 Soothing Strategies

For many women, breasts are a source of sensual pleasure. For breast-feeding mothers, they are a way of nurturing a new life. But at certain times in a woman's life, breasts can be uncomfortable or downright painful. They may even become the focus of worry and anxiety.

Breast discomfort is a normal part of being a woman. It is almost always not a sign of breast cancer. Breasts are mammary glands that are responsive to natural hormonal changes, especially fluctuations in estrogen, that occur at menstruation, menopause, and pregnancy. Hormonal changes can cause breasts to become hot, swollen, tender, and painful to the touch. "Breast discomfort is really common for women," says Amanda Clark, M.D., assistant professor of obstetrics and gynecology at Oregon Health Sciences University in Portland. "We see it a great deal during early pregnancy, with menstruation, and during early hormone therapy at menopause."

All of the hormonal changes that occur just before menstruation and during pregnancy prepare the woman's breasts for breast-feeding. With the onset of menstruation, estrogen levels fall and the breasts return to normal.

With pregnancy, the hormonal changes continue, and the breasts begin producing milk for the baby. Lactating breasts present their own special problems and challenges. Sometimes, a mother's milk comes in too early or too heavily and causes a painful condition called engorgement. Nursing nipples can become sore. Milk ducts may become backed up and can lead to a painful infection called mastitis. (For more information on preventing and treating discomfort associated with breast-feeding, see BREAST-FEEDING DISCOMFORT.)

During menopause, many women opt for hormone therapy to reduce menopausal symptoms such as hot flashes and to reduce their risk of developing the bone-thinning disease osteoporosis. However, it often takes a while to find just the right combination and dosage of hormones for each woman. During this period, many women experience breast discomfort.

Some women also suffer from a noncancerous breast condition such as fibrocystic breasts that can cause the breasts to feel lumpy, painful, and tender. The condition is related to monthly hormonal fluctuations. As many as 30 percent of all women suffer from fibrocystic breasts, according to Sadja Greenwood, M.D., assistant clinical professor in the Department of Obstetrics, Gynecology, and Reproductive Sciences at the University of California at San Francisco. "Fibrocystic breasts were once considered a disease," she says. "But it's very common and is considered a normal—although somewhat painful—condition."

Even young girls who are just beginning to develop breasts are subject to hormonal fluctuations and can therefore experience breast tenderness. "Breast discomfort in prepubescent young women with breast budding is normal," says Deborah Purcell, M.D., a pediatrician in private practice and past chairperson of the Department of Pediatrics at St. Vincent Hospital and Medical Center in Portland, Oregon. As odd as it may sound, "even young boys can experience some enlargement of the breasts and discomfort during this growth spurt," says Purcell.

While you can't always escape the natural fluctuations in hormones, there are things you can do to make yourself and your breasts more comfortable.

Wear a supportive bra. Breasts often swell with fluid during periods of hormonal fluctuation. Susan Woodruff, B.S.N., childbirth and parenting education coordinator at Tuality Community Hospital in Hillsboro, Oregon, advises women to wear a supportive bra, especially if their breasts are large. "You may have to wear it 24 hours a day when the breasts are tender," she says. "Try one of those soft athletic bras that provide comfort and good support."

HELLO, DOCTOR?

While some causes of breast discomfort can be effectively treated at home, see a doctor if you have any of the following symptoms:
- A lump or firmness
- Soreness in only one breast
- A change in your breast self-exam
- Nipple discharge on one side (Lactating breasts may secrete white/yellow discharge for up to a year after nursing is discontinued.)

In addition, be sure to examine your breasts monthly, regardless of whether you are having any discomfort or not. Self-examination of the breasts is an effective way to detect cancerous changes early. The best time to perform the examination is during the week following your menstrual period. If you do not know how to do a breast self-examination or are not sure if you are doing it properly, talk to your doctor.

Try cutting back on caffeine. Greenwood says that the scientific evidence is mixed about whether or not eliminating caffeine helps lumpy, fibrocystic breasts. One study, reported by the National Institutes of Health, which included more than 3,000 women, found no relationship between caffeine consumption and fibrocystic disease. On the other hand, some women have reported good results from cutting back or eliminating caffeinated coffees, teas, colas, and chocolate. Try reducing your caffeine intake to see if your breast discomfort decreases.

Cut salt. Many women are bothered by fluid retention, particularly near the time of their menstrual period, says Clark. "Avoiding salt around this time can help minimize fluid retention," she says.

Apply heat/cold packs. Woodruff says that some women find relief from painful breasts by alternating a warm heating pad and ice packs. Try using the heating pad for 30 minutes, then the ice packs for 10 minutes, then the heating pad for 30 minutes, and so on.

Try a nonprescription pain reliever. Aspirin, ibuprofen, or acetaminophen can ease the pain of premenstrual breasts, says Clark. For fibrocystic breasts, Purcell recommends ibuprofen.

Check out your cosmetics. Some herbal cosmetics and remedies, such as those made with ginseng, can have steroidal effects similar to estrogen. If you suspect that a product that you use may have such an effect, try avoiding the product temporarily to see if your condition improves.

BREAST-FEEDING DISCOMFORT

19 Ways to Beat the Breast-feeding Blues

Throughout your pregnancy, you probably fantasized about the wonderful experience breast-feeding would be for both you and your baby. All you could think about was looking down into that tiny, trusting face and feeling the closeness between you and this new little being. So naturally, when it finally came time to put baby to breast, you were excited. But now, you're in agony. Your nipples are sore, cracked, and bleeding. If your milk has already come in, your breasts may be painfully swollen. The milk may not flow when you need it to and may seem to flow uncontrollably when you most wish it wouldn't (like when you're standing in line at the grocery store). So where are those tender, happy moments you've seen in the magazine and television advertisements?

Well, hang in there. Those moments do actually exist, just not right off the bat. The problem is, many mothers give up breast-feeding in frustration because they don't realize that things will get better with time. They also don't realize that there are things they can do to decrease breast-feeding discomfort.

As far as what causes breast-feeding pain, it depends on what part of the breast you are talking about. Nipple pain is most often caused by the baby latching on to the nipple incorrectly. "If the baby doesn't latch on in a way that allows the nipple to get adjusted correctly in his palate, it can be very traumatic for the breast," says Phyllis Frey, A.R.N.P., a nurse practitioner with Bellegrove OB-GYN, Inc., in Bellevue, Washington. In addition, she notes, "American women tend to experience more nipple discomfort than foreign women because we always wear bras to protect that sensitive skin. Foreign women, however, go braless more often and sunbathe topless, which toughens the nipples." Pre-existing conditions, such as inverted nipples or nipple sensitivity that developed during the pregnancy, can also cause problems.

Pain in the fleshy part of the breast is most often caused by engorgement of the breast with milk when the milk first comes in. Engorgement may also make the breasts feel sore in between feedings.

While you can't escape all initial discomfort from breast-feeding, there are some tips and techniques you can use to prevent or alleviate much of the pain.

Make sure the baby latches on correctly. Despite what you may have been told, breast-feeding is a learned skill, and it takes time and practice to perfect. "If the baby is latching on at the very end of the nipple, he is really mashing his gums against that tender skin," says Raven Fox, R.N., I.B.C.L.C., a registered nurse and lactation consultant/educator at Evergreen Hospital Medical Center in Kirkland, Washington. "If this motion persists, the nipples can start to crack, bleed, and blister, all of which leaves them more vulnerable to infection," she continues. The key is to get the baby's mouth open wide, lift your breast from underneath, and pull the baby in close as quickly as possible. "You want to get the baby to close down on the areola (the darkened area around the nipple), rather than on the nipple itself. And if you bring him in too slowly, he will clamp down as soon as his lips touch the nipple," Fox explains. When the baby does close directly on the nipple, you'll know it. "You may feel a general tenderness when the baby first latches on, or you may experience a real sharp pain, almost as if someone had pinched you," she warns.

Use a prop. Place the baby on a pillow on your lap when breast-feeding. "Doing so lifts the baby up a little higher so that once on, he isn't further irritating the nipple area by tugging down on it," says Frey.

Go easy at first. "It's so exciting initially to breast-feed your baby, and you often feel you don't want to interrupt him when he's finally latched on and gulping away," says Frey. "But you will pay later," she warns. She recommends limiting the breast-feeding time for the first five days of breast-feeding. Try five minutes on each breast at first. If you don't notice yourself getting tender, you can increase that time rather quickly.

Then, nurse, nurse, nurse. Once your milk comes in, let the baby nurse as long as he or she wants to. "Babies go through a marathon nursing period right as their mother's milk is coming in, and we recommend letting the baby nurse constantly during this 12- to 24-hour period. Just get it into your head that this will be your sole job for the next 24 hours," advises Fox. "We're finding that women who resign themselves to doing this are totally missing that initial engorgement period because the baby is helping to siphon off all of the excess milk the body initially produces." After all, the body automatically makes enough milk for twins; it then gradually lowers its milk production to meet one baby's needs if there is no twin. Fox goes on to say that if you trap yourself into feeding the baby every three to four hours and letting the baby sleep as long as he or she wants, your milk will come in and make your breasts look and feel as if they're going to explode. "The engorgement period should only last 36 to 48 hours, but the pain makes it seem like five years," she says.

Don't reach for the pump. If you do get engorged, resist the urge to express milk with a manual or electric breast pump. Unfortunately, the body doesn't know the difference between a pump and a baby's mouth. Whenever milk is drawn from the breast, the body thinks it's being used by the baby and makes more to compensate for that loss. So the more you pump, the more milk your body produces. "In essence, using a breast pump introduces a twin to your body," says Fox. The only time this advice wouldn't apply is when you are on a trip away from your baby and want to continue nursing regularly when you return, or when your baby is ill and his or her appetite

TREATING BREAST INFECTIONS

Cracked and bleeding nipples brought on by those first few days of breast-feeding can leave you vulnerable to breast infection, or mastitis. While rarely serious, mastitis can be quite painful and cannot be cured without antibiotics.

According to Raven Fox, R.N., I.B.C.L.C., signs that you may have mastitis include a reddened area on the fleshy part of the breast that is painful to the touch and ranges from the size of a quarter to the whole side of the breast, a fever of up to 102 degrees Fahrenheit, general achiness, and chills. You may have one or all of these symptoms. They tend to come on rapidly.

While you will need to see a doctor if you suspect a breast infection, you should do a few things on your own.

Continue nursing, starting with the infected breast each time. It helps clear the infection and will not hurt the baby. "The milk is absolutely not infected. It is the area around the milk duct that is infected," stresses Fox. She recommends nursing at least every two to three hours, and more often if the baby is willing.

Prior to nursing, pack the breast in heat. Use a warm towel with a plastic bag over it to maintain heat. "Then massage and stroke the breast from the fleshy part down to the nipple, focusing especially on that sore spot," says Phyllis Frey, A.R.N.P.

Get in bed. Go on full bed rest. Take care of yourself and let everyone else nurture you while you get over the infection. Usually, it takes only about 24 to 36 hours for the pain to pass. But Fox stresses the importance of continuing the antibiotics throughout their full 10- to 14-day course, even if you feel better.

Other problems that can cause discomfort include yeast infections in the nipple and clogged milk ducts. "Yeast infections can cause ongoing discomfort in the nipple and need to be diagnosed and treated by your doctor," says Frey. Clogged ducts, on the other hand, usually resolve within 24 hours. They are marked by a hard, uncomfortable lump in the fleshy part of the breast. It can be very tender to the touch but isn't usually accompanied by a fever. To relieve the pain, pack the breast in heat before feedings, get the baby to nurse on the infected breast first, and massage the hard spot the whole time the baby is nursing.

"If the milk is locked in the duct for more than 24 hours, it can start leaking into the breast tissue and leave a moist breeding ground for bacteria," cautions Frey. "And once it becomes infected, it is a hot spot that hurts all of the time." Fox adds that the pattern tends to be sore nipples, engorgement, clogged ducts, and mastitis. Solving the first two will usually prevent the third.

is temporarily down. In these instances, you would want to pump at the baby's normal feeding times to keep up your milk supply.

Air them out. Try to expose your nipples to air whenever possible to help toughen them up. "If you finish nursing and immediately put your bra back on with a nursing pad in it, you're likely to get some milk leakage that will wet the pad and keep moisture against the nipple," says Frey. "This further softens the nipple, which is not what you want." Instead, she suggests keeping your bra flaps open (on a nursing bra) or going braless under a light T-shirt for at least 15 minutes after feeding. If you were planning to nap after a feeding, you might consider napping braless, as well.

Stand in a warm shower. This causes some milk to drip from the breasts, which can relieve some of the pressure, according to Frey. But unlike pumping the breast, this technique doesn't cause the body to produce more milk. It just provides welcome relief as long as the water is hitting directly on the breasts. "Another way to get similar relief is to fill the sink with warm water, take your bra off, lean over the sink, and splash the water up over your breasts," says Fox.

Try "cold storage." Between feedings, pack your breasts in ice, and wear a bra to hold the ice in place. "My favorite way to do this is to freeze four Ziploc bags of unpopped popcorn. The popcorn holds the cold much longer than the frozen peas and carrots many people use, and it doesn't get mushy. It also molds to the shape of your breasts so that you don't have big, bulky ice cubes lying on you," says Fox. "Usually, engorgement in between feedings lasts no more than seven to ten days after the baby's birth. This is because the mother's milk production and the baby's milk consumption are still balancing out," explains Harold Zimmer, M.D., an obstetrician and gynecologist in private practice in Bellevue, Washington.

Warm up for feedings. Fifteen minutes before feeding your baby, warm up your breasts. "Soak a bath towel in hot

TAKING THE PAIN OUT OF WEANING

Once you get through the initial discomfort of breast-feeding, nursing becomes easy and relatively painless until that fateful day when you decide it is time to wean your baby off of the breast. In addition to producing some emotional discomfort, weaning can cause physical pain. As you decrease feedings, it takes a little time for the body to catch on and produce less milk in response, so the engorgement of those early days often returns.

"Every expert is a little different in terms of their advice on how to best wean a baby," says Harold Zimmer, M.D. "Some advise you to go 'cold turkey' and some advise you to truly wean," he continues. For Mom, it is a little more comfortable to do it gradually, but some babies will decide to wean themselves and will abruptly reject the breast for good. "Generally, trying to drop one feeding about every two days is what I recommend," says Zimmer. "And the last feedings to be dropped should be the first one in the morning and the last one at night because the baby tends to be most attached to breast-feeding at these times," he explains. It is also important to never drop two feedings in a row. In other words, if you typically breast-feed your baby twice in the morning, twice in the afternoon, and twice in the evening, avoid dropping one morning feeding one day and another morning feeding two days later. Instead, try dropping one morning feeding, then an afternoon feeding, then an evening feeding.

As far as the pain of engorgement that can result, there are a few things you can do. "Tying a towel or Ace bandage around your breasts can help decrease your milk supply, because the extra pressure collapses the glands so that they can't hold as much milk," says Zimmer. "Applying ice packs to the breasts decreases circulation and further reduces the degree of engorgement and swelling," he continues. And once you have started to wean, he gives his OK to taking aspirin. "Aspirin is a good anti-inflammatory and can relieve some of the discomfort of engorgement," he says.

Whatever you do, avoid any extra stimulation to the breasts during weaning. "Anything that stimulates the breasts will promote more milk production," warns Zimmer.

water, wring it out, and place it across your breasts with a plastic garbage bag over it to maintain the heat a little longer," advises Fox. Then take it off and massage the breast from the fleshy part down to the nipple to en-

HELLO, DOCTOR?

If none of these tips seems to help much, it's time to see your doctor to rule out the possibility of a breast infection. In addition, your local chapter of the La Leche League and most hospital maternity wards can offer over-the-phone answers to your breast-feeding questions.

courage the release of milk into the nipple. "Latching your baby onto an empty nipple can hurt so much more than if there is milk in the nipple," says Frey.

Try the "burp and switch" strategy. Always begin a feeding on the sorest breast or the one that seems fullest. "Once the baby is latched on, let him nurse for five minutes, and then burp him and switch him to the other side for five minutes. Continue switching him every five minutes until he is finished eating," recommends Fox. This method ensures that the baby drains both breasts sufficiently, rather than tanking up on one and leaving the other ready to explode.

Try some tea. Placing warm tea bags on your nipples a few times a day is one of the best home remedies around for nipple discomfort, according to Zimmer. Fox stresses that it has to be black tea, as opposed to chamomile or yellow tea, because black tea contains tannin, and the tannic acid is what soothes and toughens up the nipples. Soak the tea bags in warm water for a few minutes, squeeze them out, and place them on the nipples for ten minutes.

Massage the nipples with an ice cube. "This will numb the painful area and give you some temporary relief," says Zimmer. But he goes on to say that once the numbness wears off, the nipples will be just as painful as before. "It is not a healing remedy as much as it is a relief mechanism," he explains.

Wear a well-supporting bra. "You want to avoid as much additional trauma to the breasts as possible, and this is one way to protect them somewhat," says Zimmer.

Take acetaminophen if you develop a fever. It is very common to develop a low-grade fever as high as 100.2 to 100.6 degrees Fahrenheit, according to Fox. Acetaminophen should help to lower it and make you feel a little better. Be sure to check with your doctor, however, before taking any medication while you are nursing.

Take ibuprofen if you feel achy. "It is also not uncommon to feel as if a truck has run over you," warns Fox. If this is the case, ibuprofen should help relieve some of the aches and discomfort. Once again, however, check with your doctor before taking any medications.

CHAPPED LIPS

7 Tips for Smoother Lips

If puckering is painful and pursing is too much to bear, you're probably suffering from chapped lips. Harsh winter weather, dry indoor heat, a habit of constantly licking your lips—all of these factors can help dry out the skin of your lips by causing the moisture in the skin to evaporate. The result: rough, cracked, sensitive lips that leave you little to smile about.

Protecting your lips from chapping is not only important for appearance and comfort, but for health. Cold sores, bacterial infections, and other problems are more likely to strike lips that are already damaged by chapping. Here's what you can do to keep your lips soft and moist:

Don't lick your lips. The repeated exposure to water actually robs moisture from the lips, causing them to become dry. "People feel better if they lick their lips, but it just aggravates the problem," says Paul Lazar, M.D., professor of clinical dermatology at Northwestern University School of Medicine in Chicago.

Use a lip balm. Numerous products are available over the counter. Pick one that you like so you'll use it frequently. Most lip balm products are waxy or greasy and work by sealing in moisture with a protective barrier.

Try petrolatum. Plain old petrolatum is good, too, says Jerome Z. Litt, M.D., assistant clinical professor of dermatology at Case Western Reserve University School of Medicine in Cleveland.

Screen out the sun. The sun's ultraviolet rays can damage and dry the sensitive skin on your lips. Indeed, the lips are a common site for skin cancer. "Your lips don't contain melanin [the pigment, or coloring, that can help protect skin from the sun] and they sunburn easier," points out Ruby Ghadially, M.D., assistant clinical professor in the Department of Dermatology at the University of California at San Francisco. Certain skin cancers that appear on the lips may be more serious and more likely to spread, she says. So if you'll be out in the sun, use a lip balm that contains sunscreen. Choose a product that has a sun protection factor (SPF) of 15 or higher.

Wear lipstick. "If you look at old men and old women, you'll see a difference in their lips, especially the lower," says Albert M. Kligman, M.D., Ph.D., emeritus professor of dermatology at the University of Pennsylvania School of Medicine in Philadelphia. He attributes that difference to the "moderately helpful" properties of lipstick in moisturizing and protecting against the sun's ultraviolet rays. Be careful of cosmetics made outside of the United States, however, since the purity of such products may vary.

Check out your toothpaste. An allergy—to your toothpaste or mouthwash—could be to blame for the rough, red skin on your lips, says Litt. Try switching brands of toothpaste and going without the mouthwash for a few days to see if the problem clears. In addition, be sure to rinse well after brushing.

Watch what passes between them. When your lips are chapped, they're more sensitive, and certain foods can irritate them further. Lazar recommends holding off on pepper, mustard, barbecue sauce, orange juice (and other citrus juices), and alcoholic beverages to give your lips a break as they heal.

COLDS

11 Tips for Fighting the "Cold" War

Headache. Stuffy nose. Cough. Fever. Itchy eyes. Sore throat. Muscle aches. If you're like most people, you know the symptoms of the common cold all too well. Although Americans spend more than $5 billion annually on doctor visits and cold remedies—everything from tissues and vitamin C to over-the-counter decongestants and herb teas—there is no cure for the common cold.

Colds, also called upper respiratory infections, are caused by hundreds of different viruses, according to David N. Gilbert, M.D., director of the Department of Medical Education at Providence Medical Center in Portland, Oregon. "But we don't have any drugs that can kill or inhibit these viruses," he says. "We have to depend on the body's natural defenses."

During a cold, virus particles penetrate the mucous layer of the nose and throat and attach themselves to cells there. The viruses punch holes in the cell membranes, allowing viral genetic material to enter the cells. Within a short time, the virus takes over and forces the cells to produce thousands of new virus particles.

In response to this viral invasion, the body marshals its defenses: The nose and throat release chemicals that spark the immune system; injured cells produce chemicals called prostaglandins, which trigger inflammation and attract infection-fighting white blood cells; tiny blood vessels stretch, allowing spaces to open up to allow blood fluid (plasma) and specialized white cells to enter the infected area; the body temperature rises, enhancing the immune response; and histamine is released, increasing the production of nasal mucus in an effort to trap the viral particles and remove them from the body.

As the battle against the cold virus rages on, the body counterattacks with its heavy artillery—specialized white blood cells called monocytes and lymphocytes; interferon, often called the "body's own antiviral drug"; and 20 or more proteins that circulate in the blood plasma and coat the viruses and infected cells, making it easier for the white blood cells to identify and destroy them.

The symptoms you experience as a cold are actually the body's natural immune response. In fact, says Michael Castleman, author of *Cold Cures,* by the time you feel like you're coming down with a cold, you've likely already had it for a day and a half.

Many people believe the old adage, "Do nothing and your cold will last seven days. Do everything and it will last a week." While we may not be able to cure the common cold, the simple self-care techniques that follow can help you feel more comfortable and speed healing.

Drink plenty of fluids. "Fluids keep the mucus thin," says Gilbert. Donald Girard, M.D., head of the Division of General Internal Medicine at Oregon Health Sciences University in Portland, agrees. "Colds can make you somewhat dehydrated and you don't even know it," says Girard. Drink at least eight ounces of fluid every two hours.

Cook up some chicken soup. One of the most beneficial hot fluids you can consume when you have a cold is chicken soup. It was first prescribed for the common cold by rabbi and physician Moses Maimonides in twelfth-century Egypt and has been a favorite folk remedy ever since. In 1978, Marvin Sackner, M.D., of Mount Sinai Hospital in Miami Beach, Florida, included chicken soup in a test of the effects of sipping hot and cold water on the clearance of mucus. Chicken soup placed first, hot water second, and cold water a distant third. Sackner's work has since been replicated by other researchers. While doctors aren't sure exactly why chicken soup helps clear nasal passages, they agree "it's just what the doctor ordered."

Rest. Doctors disagree about whether or not you should take a day or two off from work when you come down with a cold. However, they do agree that extra rest helps. Staying away from the work site may be a good idea from a prevention standpoint, too. Your coworkers will probably appreciate your not spreading your cold virus around the office. If you do decide to stay home, forgo all those household chores. Take it easy—read a good book, watch some television, take a nap.

HELLO, DOCTOR?

While most colds can be effectively treated at home, you should call your doctor if:

• You have a headache and stiff neck with no other cold symptoms. (Your symptoms may indicate meningitis.)

• You have a headache and sore throat with no other cold symptoms. (It may be strep throat.)

• You have cold symptoms and significant pain across your nose and face that doesn't go away. (You may have a sinus infection, which requires antibiotics.)

• You have a fever above 101 degrees Fahrenheit (adults), you've taken aspirin, and the fever isn't going down.

• Your child has a fever above 102 degrees Fahrenheit.

• Your cold symptoms seem to be going away, but you suddenly develop a fever. (It may indicate pneumonia, which is more likely to set in toward the end of a cold.)

• You have a "dry" cough—one that doesn't bring up phlegm—for more than ten days.

• You cough up blood.

Girard adds that you should skip your normal exercise routine when you've got a cold. In fact, he says, if you're feeling pretty bad, you should just head for bed.

Stay warm. "I usually recommend people stay indoors and stay warm when they have a cold," says Girard. If nothing else, staying warm may make you feel more comfortable, especially if you have a fever.

Use a saltwater wash. The inflammation and swelling in the nose during a cold is caused by molecules called cytokines, or lymphokines, which are made by the lymphocytes, explains Stephen R. Jones, M.D., chief of medicine at Good Samaritan Hospital and Medical Center in Portland, Oregon. "Recent evidence has shown that if we can wash out those cytokines, it reduces the swelling and fluid production." Jones recommends filling a clean nasal-spray bottle with dilute salt water (one level teaspoon salt to one quart water) and spraying each nostril three or four times. Repeat five to six times per day.

Gargle. Girard says gargling with warm salt water (a quarter teaspoon salt in four ounces warm water) every one to two hours can soothe your sore throat. "Salt water is an astringent that is very soothing to the inflamed tissues, and it tends to loosen mucus," he says.

Consider vitamin C. Although studies suggest that vitamin C may boost the body's immune system, the use of this vitamin in treating colds is still controversial. Many physicians don't recommend vitamin C as a cold remedy. Others, including cold researcher Elliot Dick, Ph.D., chief of the Respiratory Virus Research Laboratory at the University of Wisconsin–Madison, have found that taking 2,000 milligrams or more of vitamin C daily can lessen the severity of cold symptoms.

If you do decide to try boosting your vitamin C intake during a cold, don't overdo it. While vitamin C has been found to be relatively safe at doses of up to 10,000 milligrams per day, some people find vitamin C causes diarrhea at or above the 10,000-milligram level. Perhaps the safest way to get more vitamin C is to choose vitamin C-rich foods more often. For example, since you'll need to increase your fluid intake while you have a cold, fill some of that requirement with orange juice.

Vaporize it. The steam from a vaporizer can loosen mucus, especially if the sputum is thick, says Girard. It may also raise the humidity in the immediate area slightly, which may make you feel more comfortable.

Stop smoking. "Smokers have colds longer in duration than nonsmokers," says Gilbert. "If you chronically irritate the bronchial tubes while you have a cold, you're more likely to develop a complication like pneumonia."

In addition to irritating the throat and the bronchial tubes, smoking has been shown to depress the body's immune system. Since you have to depend on your own immune system rather than medicine to cure your cold, you'll want it to be in the best condition possible in order to wage the "cold" war.

Stay away from "hot toddies." While a hot alcoholic beverage might sound good when you're feeling achy and

WHAT ABOUT "COLD MEDICINES?"

Modern medicine doesn't have any medication that is effective against viruses, including the more than 100 viruses that can cause the common cold. Antibiotics, such as penicillin, don't work against cold viruses. "The first thing you shouldn't do," says David N. Gilbert, M.D., "is go to the doctor's office and get a penicillin shot. They're ineffective, expensive, and they expose you to unnecessary side effects."

OK, if the doctor can't help, what about all those "cold remedies" touted on television and radio? Surely they must work.

Not really. Some cold experts believe that popular cold remedies may actually inhibit the body's immune responses as they suppress cold symptoms. All of your cold symptoms are part of your body's natural response in its battle against the viral invaders. To suppress them may actually delay recovery.

For example, cold experts say a mild fever—below 102 degrees Fahrenheit—enhances the body's ability to fight the cold virus. Gilbert, therefore, suggests forgoing aspirin and acetaminophen to lower a mild fever. (If you're over 60, have heart disease, or have any immune-compromising health condition, however, contact your physician at the first sign of a fever.)

Another example of potentially counterproductive cold remedies is antihistamines, which are common ingredients in multisymptom cold formulas. Antihistamines stop the runny nose, but they may do more harm than good. "Antihistamines dry up mucous membranes, which are already irritated," says Gilbert. "They thicken the nasal mucus so you feel like you need more decongestant, and they can cause an irritated cough."

One over-the-counter cold remedy that can bring symptomatic relief is the decongestant pseudoephedrine, says Stephen R. Jones, M.D. "This ingredient effectively shuts down the swelling and fluid production and promotes drainage," he says. (People with high blood pressure or heart disease, however, should avoid this drug.) Cough syrups that contain glyceryl guaiacolate (but not dextromethorphan) can help loosen thick sputum, making it easier to cough up, according to Donald Girard, M.D.

If you think you need over-the-counter remedies to cope with your cold, most authorities recommend single-action remedies rather than the "shotgun" approach of multisymptom products. Most people get their cold symptoms serially—sore throat first, cough last. But multisymptom cold remedies say they cure all your cold symptoms at once, even the ones you don't have. Why take drugs and risk their side effects when you don't need them?

stuffy, Gilbert says it increases mucous membrane congestion. "If you want to minimize your discomfort," he says, "stay away from alcohol."

Maintain a positive attitude. Although mind-body science is in its infancy, some researchers suggest that a positive I-can-beat-this-cold attitude may actually stimulate the immune system. "If you give up, so does your immune system," says Castleman. "Buoyancy and self-confidence help rev up the immune system or at least keep it from collapsing while it fights your cold."

Jones isn't as convinced about the connection between the mind and the immune system. He says the evidence directly linking one's thoughts with immunity is "interesting, but inconclusive." But, he admits, "a positive attitude is always best and certainly couldn't hurt your cold."

CONSTIPATION

11 Ways to Keep Things Moving

Irregularity is one of those things that no one likes to talk about. It's personal and, well, a little embarrassing. But if you're one of the millions of people who's ever been constipated, you know it can put a real damper on your day.

The first thing to realize when you're talking about constipation is that "regularity" is a relative term. Everyone has his or her own natural rhythm. Ask four people to define regularity, and you're likely to get at least four different answers. Normal bowel habits can span anywhere from three bowel movements a day to three a week, according to Marvin Schuster, M.D., professor of medicine with a joint appointment in psychiatry at Johns Hopkins University School of Medicine and chief of the Division of Digestive Diseases at Francis Scott Key Medical Center, both in Baltimore.

"One of the most common forms of constipation is imaginary or misconceived constipation," says Schuster. It's based on the idea that if you don't have the "magical" one bowel movement a day, then something's wrong. Constipation has a lot to do with a person's comfort level, says Peter Banks, M.D., director of Clinical Gastroenterology Service at Brigham and Women's Hospital and lecturer on medicine at Harvard Medical School, both in Boston. People who are constipated often strain a lot in the bathroom, produce unusually hard stools, and feel gassy and bloated.

Schuster calls it "constipation" if you have fewer than three bowel movements a week or if you experience a marked change in your normal bowel patterns. A sudden change in bowel habits merits a visit to your doctor to rule out any more serious underlying problems (see "Hello, Doctor?"). But for the occasional bout of constipation, here are some tips to put you back on track:

Get moving. Exercise seems not only to boost your fitness but to promote regularity as well. "The thinking is that lack of activity puts the bowels to rest," says Banks. That may partially explain why older people, who may be more sedentary, and those who are bedridden are prone to becoming constipated. "We encourage people to get up and be more active," says Banks. So gear up and get moving. You don't have to run a marathon; a simple walking workout doesn't take much time and can be very beneficial. When it comes to regularity, even a little exercise is better than none at all.

Raise your glass. Drinking an adequate amount of liquids may help to alleviate constipation or prevent it from happening in the first place. The reason for this is simple. "If you dehydrate yourself or drink too little fluid, that will dry out your stool as well and make it hard to pass," says Schuster.

On the other hand, some people have the misconception that if you drink far more than you need, you can treat constipation. Schuster disagrees, saying the excess fluid will just get urinated out.

To achieve a balanced intake of liquids, a good rule of thumb is to drink eight cups of fluid a day, says Mindy Hermann, R.D., a registered dietitian and spokesperson for the American Dietetic Association. (This rule of thumb doesn't apply, however, if you have a kidney or liver

HELLO, DOCTOR?

Constipation can be a symptom of a more serious problem, such as an underactive thyroid, irritable bowel syndrome, or cancer, to name a few. See your doctor if you have any of these symptoms:

- A major change in your bowel pattern
- Constipation lasting for several weeks or longer
- Blood in your stool
- Severe pain during bowel movements
- Unusual stomach distention

problem or any other medical condition that may require restricting your intake of fluid.) Drink even more when it's hot or when you're exercising. Hermann suggests that athletes weigh themselves before and after a workout. Any weight lost during the activity reflects water loss. To replace it, they should drink two cups of liquid for every lost pound of body weight.

For those who are constipated, all liquids are not created equal. Avoid drinking a lot of coffee or other caffeinated drinks, urges Elyse Sosin, R.D., a registered dietitian and the supervisor of clinical nutrition at Mount Sinai Medical Center in New York. Caffeine acts as a diuretic, taking fluid out of your body when you want to retain it. She suggests sticking with water, seltzer, juice, or milk instead.

Don't fight the urge. Often, because people are busy or have erratic schedules or because they don't want to use public bathrooms, they suppress the urge to have a bowel movement. "If they do this over a period of time, it can block the urge so it doesn't come," explains Schuster. If at all possible, heed the call when you feel it.

Take advantage of an inborn reflex. As babies, we're all born with a reflex to defecate a short time after we're fed, says Schuster. With socialization, we learn to control our bladders and bowels and we inhibit this reflex. Schuster suggests that you try to revive this reflex by choosing one mealtime a day and trying to have a movement after it. "Very often, people can program the colon to respond to that meal." Schuster says that this works better with younger people than with the elderly.

Know your medications. A number of prescription and over-the-counter medications can cause constipation. If you are currently taking any medication, you might want to ask your doctor or pharmacist whether it could be causing your constipation. Among the drugs that can cause constipation are calcium-channel blockers taken for high blood pressure, beta-blockers, some antidepressants, narcotics and other pain medications, antihistamines (to a lesser degree), certain decongestants, and some antacids. Antacids that contain calcium or aluminum are binding and can cause constipation. When choosing an antacid, Schuster suggests you keep in mind that the names of most of those with aluminum start with the letter "a." Those that start with the letter "m" contain magnesium, which does not constipate. If you are unsure, check the label or ask your pharmacist.

Bulk up. Many times, adding fiber or roughage to your diet is all that's needed to ensure regularity. Fiber, the indigestible parts of plant foods, adds mass to the stool and stimulates the colon to push things along. Fiber is found in fruits, vegetables, grains, and beans. Meats, chicken, fish, and fats come up empty-handed in the fiber category. The current recommendations for daily dietary fiber are 20 to 35 grams. "Most people eat between 10 and 15 grams," says Hermann. So there's plenty of room for improvement. Fiber supplements may be helpful, but most doctors and dietitians agree that it's preferable to get your fiber from food (see "Laxative Alert").

Add fiber slowly. People assimilate high-fiber foods into their diet more easily if they do it gradually. "You need to add one high-fiber food at a time, start with small amounts, and wait a couple of days before adding something else so you don't throw your system into chaos," says Hermann. Sosin agrees and also stresses the need to "drink an adequate amount of fluids with the fiber."

Eat at least five servings of fruits and vegetables daily. Select a variety of fruits and vegetables, recommends

LAXATIVE ALERT

Laxatives seem like an easy solution for constipation woes, but they can cause many more problems than they solve. Indeed, these tablets, gums, powders, suppositories, and liquids can be habit forming and produce substantial side effects if used incorrectly.

Laxatives work in many different ways, and "each one has its problems," says Marvin Schuster, M.D. Some lubricate, others soften the stools, some draw water into the bowel, and still others are bulk forming. One real danger is that people can become dependent on them, needing ever-increasing amounts to do the job. Eventually, some types of laxatives can damage the nerve cells of the colon until the person can't evacuate anymore. Some laxatives inhibit the absorption or effectiveness of drugs. Those with a mineral-oil base can prevent the absorption of vitamins A, D, K, and E. Still others can damage and inflame the lining of the intestine.

"I think laxatives ought to be avoided if at all possible and only used under a doctor's care," says Schuster. In the long run, you'll be much better off to depend on exercise, adequate fluid intake, and a high-fiber diet to keep you regular.

Hermann, some that are high in fiber and others that aren't so high. Potatoes (white and sweet), apples, berries, apricots, peaches, pears, oranges, prunes, corn, peas, carrots, tomatoes, broccoli, and cauliflower are all good choices.

Eat 6 to 11 servings of grain products daily. That's in addition to the five servings of fruits and vegetables just mentioned. Grain products include cereals, breads, and starchy vegetables (such as corn, green peas, potatoes, and lima beans). "I tell people to start out the day with a high-fiber cereal because it's easy to do and it immediately knocks off a big chunk of the amount of fiber they should be getting during the day," says Hermann. Check the labels on cereal boxes; anything with more than five or six grams of fiber per serving qualifies as high fiber. If you don't like any so-called "high fiber" cereals, line up the boxes of cereal that you would be willing to eat and pick the one with the most fiber, suggests Hermann.

Read labels when choosing breads as well. "Just because a bread is brown doesn't mean it has a lot of fiber in it," says Hermann. Find a bread that has at least two grams of fiber per slice. Watch the portion size, too, when looking for high-fiber foods. "Sometimes they will give you a very large size that's unrealistic for one serving," says Sosin.

Bring home the beans. Dried beans and legumes—whether pinto, red, lima, navy, or garbanzo—are excellent sources of fiber. Many people don't like them because of the gassiness they may cause. Cooking beans properly can ease this problem considerably. Hermann's technique for cooking less "explosive" dried beans: Soak the beans overnight, then dump the water out. Pour new water in, and cook the beans for about 30 minutes. Throw that water out, put in new water, and cook for another 30 minutes. Drain the water out, put new water in, and finish cooking.

Cut back on refined foods. You can bump up your fiber intake by switching from refined foods to less-refined foods whenever possible. Switch from a highly processed cereal to a whole-grain cereal, move from heavily cooked vegetables to less-cooked vegetables, and choose whole-grain products over products made with white flour. A glass of orange juice, for instance, provides 0.1 gram of fiber, while eating an orange gives you 2.9 grams. And while a serving of potato chips has only 0.6 gram of fiber, a serving of popcorn supplies 2.5 grams. "As soon as you start juicing something or straining it or taking the pulp out, you're taking out the fiber," says Hermann.

CORNS AND CALLUSES
22 Steps to Relief

You may refer to your feet as tootsies or dogs, but the fact remains that feet are highly sophisticated structures. The human foot is a miracle of engineering designed to stand up under a lot of wear and tear. It's a good thing, too: Your feet are the most used and abused parts of your body. According to the American Podiatric Medical Association, the average American walks 115,000 miles in a lifetime—a distance that would take you all the way around the earth four times. Your feet support the weight of your body, plus clothing and whatever extras you might be carrying. And in an average day of walking, your feet are subjected to a force equal to several hundred tons.

Despite how well designed your feet are, however, things can go wrong. In fact, an estimated 87 percent of all American adults have some type of foot problem. Among the most common of these problems are corns and calluses.

Although both corns and calluses are patches of toughened skin that form to protect sensitive foot tissue against repeated friction and pressure, they are different in some ways. Hard corns are usually found on the tops of the toes or on the outer sides of the little toes, where the skin rubs against the shoe. Sometimes, a corn will form on the ball of the foot, beneath a callus, resulting in a sharp, localized pain with each step. Soft corns, which are moist and rubbery, form between toes, where the bones of one toe exert pressure on the bones of its neighbor. Both hard and soft corns are cone shaped, with the tip pointing into the foot (what you see is the base of the cone). When a shoe or another toe puts pressure against the corn, the tip can hit sensitive underlying tissue, causing pain.

Calluses, on the other hand, generally form over a flat surface and have no tip. They usually appear on the weight-bearing parts of the foot—the ball or the heel. Each step presses the callus against underlying tissue and may cause aching, burning, or tenderness, but rarely sharp pain.

There are some things you can do to relieve the discomfort associated with these two conditions. Try the tips that follow. If, despite trying these strategies, your corn or callus continues to cause discomfort, see a podiatrist. In addition, if you have diabetes or any other disorder that affects circulation, do not attempt to self-treat any foot problem; see your podiatrist right away.

Play detective. "Corns and calluses develop for a reason," says Suzanne M. Levine, D.P.M., a podiatrist in private practice in New York. "Abnormal amounts of dead, thickened skin form at certain spots on your feet to protect them from excess pressure and friction." Obviously, the real solution to corns and calluses is to track down and eliminate whatever is causing the pressure and friction. "The place to start is with your shoes," advises Levine. See "If the Shoe Fits . . ." for tips on choosing shoes.

Trim those toenails. Toenails are designed to protect the toes from injury. However, the pressure of a shoe on a toenail that is too long can force the joint of the toe to push up against the shoe, forming a corn. To take the pressure off, keep your toenails trimmed. Cut each toenail straight across so that it doesn't extend beyond the tip of the toe. Then, file each toenail to smooth any rough edges.

Take a soak. While eliminating the source of the problem is essential, sometimes you need immediate relief from the sharp pain of a corn. Levine suggests soaking the affected foot in a solution of Epsom salts and warm water, then smoothing on a moisturizing cream, and wrapping the foot in a plastic bag. Keep the bag on for a couple of hours. Then remove the bag and gently rub the corn in a sideways motion with a pumice stone. "This will provide temporary relief—and I stress temporary," says Levine.

Ice a hard corn. If a hard corn is so painful and swollen that you can't even think of putting a shoe on your foot, apply ice to the corn to help reduce some of the swelling and discomfort.

Don't cut. There are a myriad of paring and cutting items to remove corns and calluses available in your local drugstore or variety store, but you should ignore them all, in the best interest of your feet. "Cutting corns is always dangerous," says Mary Papadopoulos, D.P.M., a podiatrist in private practice in Alexandria, Virginia. "You can expose yourself to an infection, or you may cause bleeding that is not easily stopped." In addition, be sure to read "Over-the-Counter Corn and Callus Removers" on page 70 if you're thinking of trying such products.

IF THE SHOE FITS . . .

"**W**hen corns and calluses form, the real underlying problem is one of mechanics—the foot inside the shoe is not functioning properly. But poor-fitting shoes may precipitate the problem," says Joseph C. D'Amico, D.P.M.

Here are some guidelines to getting a better fit:

• Have the salesclerk measure each foot twice before you buy any pair of shoes. Don't ask for a certain size just because it's the one you have always worn; the size of your feet changes as you grow older.

• Be sure to try on both the left and the right shoe. Stand during the fitting process, and check to see that there is adequate space (three-eighths to one-half inch) for your longest toe at the end of each shoe. Remember, your longest toe may not be your big toe; in some people, the second toe extends the farthest. Likewise, your feet may not be the exact same size. If one foot is slightly larger than the other, buy the shoes for the larger foot and use padding, if necessary, for a better fit on the smaller foot.

• Make sure that the shoe fits snugly at the heel.

• Make sure the ball of your foot fits snugly into the widest part of the shoe—called the ball pocket.

• Shop for shoes at the end of the day, when your feet are likely to be slightly swollen.

• Walk around the store in the shoes to make sure they fit and feel right as you stride along.

• Don't buy shoes that feel too tight, expecting them to stretch out. If they don't feel right in the store, they will never fit comfortably. They should not need to be stretched.

• If you are not sure about the fit, check into the store's refund policy. If possible, take the shoes home, wear them on a rug for an hour, and if they don't feel good, take them back.

• When buying shoes for everyday use, look for ones with fairly low heels.

• Make sure the material of the upper is soft and pliable.

• Have several different pairs of shoes so that you do not wear the same pair day after day.

You may discover, as most people do, that your left and right foot are not exactly the same size. Or you may have a high instep, a plump foot, or especially long toes. While these characteristics may make it somewhat difficult to step into every pair of shoes you try on, they do not mean that you must resign yourself to never finding a pair of shoes that fit. All it takes is a little time and the determination to walk in comfort.

CORNS AND CALLUSES

Soft step it. "You can give yourself temporary relief from corns and calluses with shielding and padding," says Joseph C. D'Amico, D.P.M., a podiatrist in private practice in New York. What you want the padding to do is transfer the pressure of the shoe from a painful spot to one that is free of pain. Nonmedicated corn pads, for example, surround the corn with material that is higher than the corn itself, thus protecting the corn from contact with the shoe.

A similar idea applies when padding a callus. Cut a piece of moleskin (available at your local drugstore or camping supply store) into two half-moon shapes and place the pieces on opposite sides of the area to protect it.

OVER-THE-COUNTER CORN AND CALLUS REMOVERS

Salicylic acid is the only over-the-counter drug that is safe and effective for treating calluses and hard corns, according to the Food and Drug Administration (FDA). For medicated disks, pads, or plasters, the recommended concentration of salicylic acid is 12 percent to 40 percent. A concentration of 12 percent to 17.6 percent is recommended for liquid forms.

Many podiatrists, however, advise against the use of these products as home remedies, mainly because the active ingredient is an acid that can burn healthy skin as well as the dead skin of a callus or corn. If you do decide to try one of these products, follow the package directions carefully and be sure to apply the product only to the area of the corn or callus, avoiding the surrounding healthy tissue (one way to do this is to spread petrolatum in a ring shape around the corn or callus). If your corn or callus does not improve within two weeks, stop using the product and see a podiatrist. If you are diabetic or have any medical condition that hinders circulation, do not try one of these products at all; see a podiatrist at the first sign of any foot problem.

The following ingredients are not generally recognized as being safe and effective for removing corns and calluses, according to the FDA: iodine, ascorbic acid, acetic acid, allantoin, belladonna, chlorobutanol, diperodon hydrochloride, ichthammol, methylbenzethonium chloride, methyl salicylate, panthenol, phenyl salicylate, and vitamin A.

Separate your piggies. To relieve soft corns that form between toes, keep the toes separated with lamb's wool or cotton. A small, felt pad, like those for hard corns, may also be used for this purpose.

Baby your soft corn. In addition to separating your toes, sprinkle a little cornstarch or baby powder between them to help absorb moisture.

Mix your own callus concoction. For calluses, Levine suggests mixing up your own callus softener. Make a paste using five or six aspirin tablets and a tablespoon of lemon juice, apply it to the callus, wrap your foot in a plastic bag, and wrap a warm towel around the bag. Wait ten minutes, then unwrap the foot and gently rub the callus with a pumice stone.

Invite your feet to tea. Soaking your feet in chamomile tea that has been thoroughly diluted has a soothing effect and, according to Levine, will help dry out sweaty feet (excessive moisture can contribute to foot problems). The chamomile will stain your feet, but the stain can be easily removed with soap and water.

Coat your feet. If you expect to be doing an unusual amount of walking or running, coat your toes with a little petroleum jelly to reduce friction.

DENTURE DISCOMFORT

9 Ways to Stop Denture Discomfort

Dentures have come a long way since the wooden teeth worn by George Washington. But, as anyone who has worn them can attest, dentures can cause discomfort. There are two times when dentures often cause discomfort—during the initial "adjustment" phase, when dentures are new, and after several years of wearing, when dentures may stop fitting properly.

Most people become accustomed to their new dentures within a short time. However, at first, you may have difficulty

HELLO, DOCTOR?

While some denture discomforts can be handled at home, Jack W. Clinton, D.M.D., says you should see your dentist if:

• You develop soreness that doesn't improve within a week.

• You have an area on the gum that bleeds spontaneously or is filled with pus.

• There's extra tissue growing, particularly between the upper lip and the gum.

• You have a white sore for more than one week.

• You have a sore that doesn't heal completely within 10 to 14 days.

talking and eating. You may find the dentures tend to "slip," or you may develop sore spots in your mouth.

Even people who have had dentures for years sometimes develop problems with them, usually problems related to fit. "When the teeth are extracted, the dentures sit on the bony ridge that's left," says Sandra Hazard, D.M.D., a managing dentist with Willamette Dental Group, Inc., in Oregon. "Without the teeth, the stimulation to the bone is gone and, over many years, the bone is reabsorbed by the body. The plastic denture, of course, stays the same but starts to fit badly."

Poor fit is probably the most common cause of denture discomfort. As the bony ridge shrinks, the dentures can slip, move around, and cause sore areas. Often, people try to refit their dentures by using commercial denture adhesives. But using too much adhesive can change the relationship of the denture to the tissue and result in more soreness. Sometimes the body itself tries to solve the ill-fitting denture problem by causing tissue to overgrow in the mouth.

While dentures will never be as comfortable as your natural teeth, there are plenty of things you can do to prevent and resolve denture discomfort:

Keep those chompers clean. When you first have your teeth extracted and your new dentures fit, it's important to keep your dentures clean, because excess bacteria can retard the gums' healing process, says Hazard.

Once you're accustomed to your dentures, it's important to clean them at least twice a day. "You can brush them with toothpaste or use a special denture cleaner," says Hazard.

Jack W. Clinton, D.M.D., associate dean of Patient Services at Oregon Health Sciences University School of Dentistry in Portland, prefers plain old soap and water to keep dentures sparkling. "Using a hand brush and soap and water works great," he says.

Brush the gums. Don't forget to brush your gums, too. "You can help maintain the health of the tissues that lie underneath the dentures by brushing the gums twice a day with a soft brush," says Ken Waddell, D.M.D., a dentist in private practice in Tigard, Oregon.

Brushing the gums, palate, and tongue not only stimulates the tissues and increases circulation, it also helps reduce bacteria and removes plaque.

Baby your mouth. At least at first, your gums will need time to adjust to the compression created by the dentures. Hazard advises patients to eat soft foods during the denture adjustment period to avoid damaging the tender tissues.

Once the gums have healed and your dentist has refit your dentures properly, you'll be able to chew more normally. But Waddell says some foods, such as apples and corn on the cob, are probably best avoided by people who wear dentures. "Advertisements show people with dentures eating all kinds of hard foods," he says. "But hard foods cause the denture to traumatize the gums and bone of the upper jaw. Cut up your apples and take the corn off the cob."

Take an over-the-counter pain reliever. During the initial break-in of your dentures, your mouth is likely to feel sore. Over-the-counter pain relievers, including aspirin, ibuprofen, and acetaminophen, can take the sting out of the pain, says Hazard.

However, if you have persistent pain or if you've worn dentures for several years and pain develops, see your dentist.

Take them out. When you develop a sore area in your mouth from dentures, Clinton says to do what comes naturally—

take them out. "If you're uncomfortable, you probably have a soft tissue injury," says Clinton. "Take the denture out and leave it out for an hour or so. In most cases, that takes care of it."

If you develop a red spot, Clinton advises going dentureless for 24 hours. Then, if it doesn't clear up or if the soreness returns when you start using your dentures again, see your dentist.

Rinse with salt water. If you're in the adjustment phase of wearing dentures or if you're a denture veteran who has developed a sore area in your mouth, Clinton advises rinsing the mouth with warm salt water (half a teaspoon of salt to four ounces of warm water). "Take out your dentures and rinse your mouth every three to four hours with the salt water," he says. "Not only does the salt water help clean out bacteria, it also helps toughen the tissue."

Try hydrogen peroxide. Rinse your mouth out once a day with oral three percent hydrogen peroxide, advises Ronald Wismer, D.M.D., past president of the Washington County Dental Society in Oregon. Mix the peroxide half and half with water, swish for 30 seconds or so (don't swallow), and spit. The hydrogen peroxide helps clean out bacteria.

Don't self-adjust. Too often, people who have worn their dentures for a while and develop a fit problem try to "adjust" their dentures themselves with a pocket knife or other tool. This can cause more harm, says Clinton, because it can break down the dentures, change the dentures' "bite," and alter how the dentures fit against the gum. Also, don't try to "fill the space" between the denture and the gum with over-the-counter adhesive. If your dentures begin to slip or don't feel like they're fitting properly, see your dentist, who can reline them.

Take time out. "I tell people their dentures should be out of their mouths half the time," says Clinton. "It gives the soft tissues time to recover."

Always take your dentures out at night, Clinton advises. "You don't sleep with your shoes on," he says. "It's the same with your dentures."

DERMATITIS AND ECZEMA
25 Ways to Fight Them

Dermatitis, which is sometimes also called eczema, can create a vicious cycle. Your skin itches, so you scratch it. It becomes red and swollen, and then tiny, red, oozing bumps appear that eventually crust over. You keep scratching because the itching is unbearable, so the rash gets even more irritated and perhaps even infected.

All too often, you don't even know what's causing the itching. It could be an allergy to the soap you use in the shower each morning. It could be irritation due to a chemical you're exposed to at work. It could be atopic eczema—a mysterious itchy rash common to people with a history of allergies and most prevalent in children.

Dermatitis is sometimes used as a catch-all term for any inflammation or swelling of the skin. The term eczema is used interchangeably with dermatitis by some experts, while others differentiate between the two as separate types of inflammation.

Regardless of what kind of dermatitis you're suffering from, some general rules apply when you're seeking relief. There are also some treatment and prevention tips that are specific to the type of dermatitis that you have. So first, we'll give you some basic strategies for relief—no matter which type of dermatitis has you scratching. Then we'll give you some specific helpful hints to protect your skin from some of the most common types of dermatitis.

RELIEF FROM THE ITCH

Determining what's causing your dermatitis is important in treating it, but if you can't think of *anything* but the itching at the moment, here are some steps you can take for fast relief.

Cool the itch and swelling. You can do this with cool compresses. Jerome Z. Litt, M.D., assistant clinical professor of dermatology at Case Western Reserve University School of Medicine in Cleveland, recommends using a folded handkerchief or a piece of bed linen folded eight layers thick. Dip the clean cloth into cool water or Burow's solution (available over the counter at your pharmacy) and

---

HELLO, DOCTOR?

When should you see a doctor for your rash? "When you feel uncomfortable with what's going on," says Paul Lazar, M.D. "Patients worry they come in too soon, when many of them come in too late because a simple problem has ended up turning into a chronic disease." He adds that if you're worried about your rash, you need to seek medical attention.

---

place it on the rash for 10 to 15 minutes every hour. Wet compresses are appropriate when weeping, oozing blisters are present; you'll actually dry up the rash by using water on it.

Litt also says whole-milk compresses are effective. "The protein in the milk helps relieve itching."

Apply calamine lotion. This old standby can help relieve the itch. Apply it in a thin layer, so that the pores aren't sealed, two to three times a day. "The problem with calamine lotion is that it's visible, so it's not very elegant," says Col. Ernest Charlesworth, M.D., assistant chief of allergy and immunology at Wilford Hall U.S. Air Force Medical Center in San Antonio. At least one manufacturer, however, has come out with a version of calamine lotion that will leave you a little less "in the pink." Check your local pharmacy.

Use an over-the-counter hydrocortisone cream. The one percent formulation of hydrocortisone is more effective, but it won't help a bacterial or fungal infection (two other common causes of skin rashes). "Hydrocortisone cream is the dermatologist's equivalent of 'take two aspirin and call me in the morning,'" says Litt. Hydrocortisone cream seems to be more effective on allergic rather than irritant dermatitis, points out Alan N. Moshell, M.D., director of the Skin Disease Program at the National Institute of Arthritis and Musculoskeletal and Skin Diseases in Bethesda, Maryland.

Stay away from products that end in "-caine." These products can often cause allergies in sensitive individuals. Charlesworth tells about a pharmacist's wife who treated a bad sunburn with a product containing benzocaine and ended up with an allergic contact dermatitis on top of her sunburn.

Don't try topical antihistamines. Again, these products can cause allergic reactions. "You should swallow an antihistamine," emphasizes Litt. "Don't ever rub it on your skin. I've seen too many horror stories—you can end up with a rash squared."

Take an oral antihistamine. Try an over-the-counter product like Benadryl to relieve itching. Such products cause drowsiness, but that may help at night when itching is most severe. If you take it during the day and it makes you drowsy, avoid driving or operating machinery.

Don't scratch. By scratching the affected area, you can break the skin and cause a secondary infection, warns Alexander A. Fisher, M.D., F.A.A.D., clinical professor of dermatology at New York University Medical Center in New York. Litt recommends rubbing the itch with your fingertips instead of scratching with your nails.

Take a soothing bath. Adding oatmeal or baking soda to bathwater will make it more soothing, says Litt, although it won't cure your rash. Buy an over-the-counter colloidal oatmeal bath treatment (the oatmeal is ground up so it dissolves better) or add a cup of baking soda to warm, not hot, bathwater.

ALLERGIC CONTACT DERMATITIS

Some people sneeze when confronted with ragweed pollen or dander from cats. And some people break out in a rash, known as allergic contact dermatitis, when confronted with substances that are normally harmless to other people, like ingredients in costume jewelry or makeup.

Confounding the issue: You have to be exposed at least once to become "sensitized," or allergic, to the substance in question. That means you might be able to wear your grandmother's ring for years before it brings on any symptoms or be able to try a new makeup for weeks before it causes a reaction.

Add to that the time delay in which a reaction occurs. An airborne allergen, like ragweed or animal dander, usually elicits sneezing or a runny nose within 15 minutes of exposure. But it may take up to 72 hours before a reaction shows up on your skin. That can make identifying the culprit pretty tough.

The most common allergen in allergic contact dermatitis is poison ivy, which can cause reactions in at least half of the people ever exposed to it.

The next most common allergen that causes this type of dermatitis is nickel, a metal commonly used in costume jewelry. Even 14-karat gold jewelry has some nickel in it. Up to ten percent of the population may suffer an allergic reaction to this metal, says Charlesworth. You're safest with 24-karat gold, which is pure gold, says Litt, or jewelry made of platinum or stainless steel.

Other possible causes of allergic contact dermatitis:

- Neomycin or benzocaine in topical anesthetics
- Leather
- Latex (most condoms and most gloves used by dentists and doctors are made of latex)
- Formaldehyde, which is used in shampoo, detergent, nail hardeners, waterless hand cleaners, and mouthwashes
- Cinnamon flavor in toothpaste and candies
- PABA, the active ingredient in some sunscreens
- Chemicals found in hair dyes
- Preservatives in cosmetics

How can you handle allergic contact dermatitis?

Ferret out the cause. If the rash recurs or won't go away, you're going to have to play detective to find out what's causing it. If you're having trouble pinning down the cause, a dermatologist or allergist can help. Either can do a test using common allergens (called a patch test) and ask you the right questions to detect the culprit. "It can be difficult," Charlesworth warns. "Some of these chemicals are present in such small amounts." What's more, we use so many different products. Paul Lazar, M.D., professor of clinical dermatology at Northwestern University School of Medicine in Chicago, points out that the average woman uses 17 different products on her scalp and head each morning.

Don't sweat it. Wearing nickel-containing jewelry in a hot, humid environment may worsen the allergy, says Charlesworth, because perspiration leaches out some of

EAR PIERCING ALERT

If you decide to get your ears pierced, make sure those first earring studs have stainless steel posts, warns Col. Ernest Charlesworth, M.D. Also make sure that the needle used is of stainless steel rather than nickel plated. Otherwise, they may contain nickel, and you'll risk becoming sensitized to this common allergen. The downside: It won't just be your earlobes that react the next time you're exposed to nickel. A watchband, ring, or belt buckle that touches the skin could set off an allergic reaction—and an itchy rash—in the future.

the nickel from jewelry. So before you start a workout or go out into the heat, take off any nickel-containing jewelry.

Don't depend on the "hypoallergenic" label. That's a "very ambiguous" term, says Charlesworth, like "low-fat" or "high-fiber" on a box of cereal. The only requirement to use the term, he says: The product has to have been tested on 200 rodent ears and not caused a reaction.

Coat nickel jewelry. Paint the surfaces that come in contact with your skin with clear nail polish.

Protect your skin. "If you're working in the garden, wear work gloves and a long-sleeved shirt," says Lazar.

IRRITANT CONTACT DERMATITIS

Some things in this world are so harsh that prolonged exposure to them can result in a rash known as irritant contact dermatitis. Numerous chemicals in industry cause problems for workers, but the household is not without its share of hazards to your skin. Soaps, detergents, oven cleaners, bathroom cleaners, and a whole multitude of products can irritate the skin by removing the skin's protective oils, explains Fisher.

What's the difference between irritant and allergic contact dermatitis? Soap, for example, can cause either one. But it's repeated exposure to soap that causes irritation, while a brief exposure to the perfume or an antibacterial agent in the soap can set off an allergic reaction, explains Moshell.

Clues to the culprit: Where is the rash on your body, and what could have touched the skin in that area?

DERMATITIS AND ECZEMA

If you suspect that an irritant has caused your red, itchy, bumpy rash, there's one very important thing you should do:

Avoid exposure to the irritant. Until you manage to do that, you'll keep subjecting the skin to the irritant, and the rash will continue. If exposure to household cleansers is the problem and it's your hands that are suffering, wear vinyl gloves, rather than those made of rubber, when handling products such as oven cleaners or when washing dishes or doing other chores that expose your hands to water, soap, and chemicals. "No one's allergic to vinyl," Fisher points out. Wearing cotton liners with the gloves will help keep perspiration from further irritating your skin, although this can be a bulky combination.

ATOPIC DERMATITIS

This one takes its name from atopy, the term for an inherited condition that can show up as dermatitis, as allergies to airborne substances such as pollens, or as asthma. If any other family members have any one of these conditions, you may be at risk for atopic dermatitis.

Infants and children are most likely to be plagued, and a majority of the cases will end by adulthood. If you or your child suffers from this chronic rash, you'll need the care of a physician, most likely a dermatologist or allergist.

It's characterized by intense and miserable itching. The key to coping with this condition is to reduce irritation to the skin, says Noreen Heer Nicol, M.S., R.N., F.N.C., a dermatology clinical specialist/nurse practitioner at National Jewish Center for Immunology and Respiratory Medicine and senior clinical instructor at the University of Colorado Health Sciences Center School of Nursing, both in Denver. Here's her advice:

Wash new clothes before wearing. This will help remove formaldehyde and other potentially irritating chemicals that are used to treat fabrics and clothing.

Rinse twice. Even if you use a mild laundry detergent, it's a good idea to rinse your clothes twice to make sure that all of the soap is removed.

Wear loose, natural-fabric clothing. You want your skin to be able to "breathe," so choose loose-fitting, open-weave, cotton or cotton-blend clothes.

Keep temperatures constant. Abrupt temperature changes—hot to cold or vice versa—can irritate the skin, so try to avoid them whenever possible. Try to maintain constant humidity levels in your home, too.

Keep your fingernails trimmed. It's hard to scratch effectively—and therefore hard to cause further damage to your sensitive skin—if your fingernails are short.

Hydrate your skin with a bath or shower. Use warm, not hot, water, and soak or shower for at least 15 or 20 minutes. Nicol recommends avoiding the use of a washcloth, except for cleaning the genital area, because it's abrasive.

Use soap only where necessary. Choose a gentle soap, such as Dove, Oiltum, Alpha Keri, Neutrogena, Purpose, or Basis; a nonsoap cleanser, such as Aveeno or Emulave; or a liquid cleaner, such as Moisturel, Neutrogena, or Dove. Rinse thoroughly, gently pat away excess moisture, and then apply moisturizer to your still-damp skin to seal in the water. Plain petrolatum is the best after-bath sealant.

Use moisturizer throughout the day. This is extremely important in atopic dermatitis, says Moshell, to prevent excessive dryness of the skin. Nicol recommends Aquaphor ointment, Eucerin cream, Moisturel cream or lotion, D.M.L. cream or lotion, Lubriderm cream or lotion, Neutrogena emulsion, Eutra, Vaseline Intensive Care lotion, or LactiCare lotion.

Protect your skin from the sun. A sunburn is only going to irritate the skin further. Whenever you go outside during the day, use a sunscreen with a sun protection factor (SPF) of 15 or more on all exposed areas of skin.

Wash after swimming. The chlorine and other chemicals found in most swimming pools can irritate the skin. So soon after you've finished your swim, take a shower or bath and use a mild soap all over. Don't forget to reapply your moisturizer as well.

Check out your diet. Some physicians believe food allergies may play some role in atopic dermatitis, while others say it hasn't been proven. If you suspect a food aggravates your rash, omit it from your diet for a few weeks. If your rash clears up, and then you eat the food again and the rash returns, you should probably eliminate it, suggests Fisher.

DIABETES

28 Ways to Live Well with Diabetes

Each day, some 12 million diabetics in this country walk a tightrope between too little sugar in the bloodstream and too much. Too little—which may come from a complication of medication—and they may quickly be overcome by dizziness, fatigue, headache, sweating, trembling, and, in severe cases, loss of consciousness and coma. Too much—which can happen after eating too much, especially if the person is older and overweight—and the person may experience weakness, fatigue, excessive thirst, labored breathing, and loss of consciousness. Left untreated, the picture is bleak: Blindness, kidney disease, blood vessel damage, infection, heart disease, nerve damage, high blood pressure, stroke, limb amputation, and coma may result.

Because the initial symptoms of diabetes (fatigue, weakness, frequent urination) are usually mild, half of all diabetics do not even realize that they have the disease. And that's a real shame, because with early diagnosis and proper treatment, the chances of living a long and productive life are higher than if the disease creeps along undetected until irreversible problems set in.

If you'd like some proof that diabetes is clearly a disease you can live with, take a look at these prolific diabetics: singer Ella Fitzgerald, actress Mary Tyler Moore, baseball Hall of Fame great Jim (Catfish) Hunter. Even before treatment was as sophisticated as it is today, author Ernest Hemingway and inventor Thomas Edison, both of whom were diabetic, managed to leave their marks on history.

If you are one of the lucky ones whose diabetes has been diagnosed by a doctor, you have an idea of what has gone awry in your body. The disorder stems from the way your body processes carbohydrates, which you take in through food. Normally, these foods are converted into a form of sugar

EARLY WARNING SIGNS

Early diagnosis and treatment is extremely important in helping diabetics live healthier, longer lives. If you notice the early warning signs listed below or suspect that you may have diabetes, see your doctor.

Some of the early warning signs of Type I diabetes are:
- Frequent urination accompanied by unusual thirst
- Extreme hunger
- Rapid weight loss with easy tiring, weakness, and fatigue
- Irritability, nausea, and vomiting

Some of the early warning signs of Type II diabetes are:
- Frequent urination accompanied by unusual thirst
- Blurred vision or any change in sight
- Tingling or numbness in the legs, feet, or fingers
- Frequent skin infection or itchy skin
- Slow healing of cuts and bruises
- Drowsiness
- Vaginitis in women
- Erectile dysfunction in men

called glucose, which floats along in the bloodstream until the pancreas, a large gland located behind the stomach, goes into action. The pancreas produces insulin, a hormone that signals body cells to soak up the glucose. Once inside the cell, the glucose is either used to produce heat or energy or is stored as fat. A person with diabetes produces little or no insulin or else becomes resistant to the hormone's action and can't compensate. Either way, the glucose can't get into the cells; it accumulates in the blood and is later expelled in the urine. In short, blood sugar rises while cells starve.

Only about one-tenth of all diabetics have the severe form of the disease, called Type I, which usually affects children and young adults and requires daily injections of insulin. Most have what doctors refer to as Type II, or adult-onset diabetes. While about one-third of Type II diabetics do require insulin to control blood sugar, and another one-third use medications to increase insulin production, the remaining Type II diabetics rely on nonmedical measures (such as diet, weight loss, and exercise) alone to control their disease. No matter which group you fall into, you can benefit from taking an active role in your treatment. But don't make a move without consulting your doctor first. He or she will call the shots; then it's up to you to carry through. Here's how:

Dish up a special diet. "The goal of dietary intervention for Type I diabetes is to help minimize short- and long-term complications by normalizing blood sugar levels. The goal of dietary intervention in Type II diabetes is to help the patient achieve and maintain normal body weight," says John Buse, M.D., Ph.D., assistant professor in the Department of Medicine, Section of Endocrinology, at the University of Chicago and director of the Endocrinology Clinic at the University of Chicago Medical Center.

Both Type I and Type II diabetics should follow the guidelines offered by the American Diabetes Association (ADA), which were revised in 1986 based on new research findings. (See "Choose One from Column A . . .")

Know your carbohydrates. The traditional dogma for diabetics was this: Avoid simple carbohydrates, or simple sugars (such as table sugar), because they raise blood sugar quickly, and choose complex carbohydrates (such as the starches and fiber found in grains, potatoes, beans, and peas), because they raise blood sugar more slowly. But this dogma has given way recently to newer rules, which really aren't rules at all in the strictest sense.

"Diabetic meal planning must account for many factors," says Harold E. Lebovitz, M.D., professor of medicine, chief of the Division of Endocrinology and Diabetes, and director of the Clinical Research Center at State University of New York Health Science Center at Brooklyn. "A food eaten alone may affect blood sugar differently than when it is eaten with another food. The same variations can be noted with cooked foods versus raw foods and even with different brands of foods. And not least, different foods affect blood sugar differently in different people."

Consequently, while complex carbohydrates like lentils, soy beans, peanuts, and kidney beans are still best for causing the slowest and lowest rise in blood sugar after a meal, present evidence suggests that sucrose (table sugar) may not be "off limits" for Type II diabetics if blood glu-

CHOOSE ONE FROM COLUMN A . . .

These recommendations should be considered "ground rules" for a Type II diabetic. Diets must be adjusted to meet individual needs, so be sure to discuss your diet with your doctor before making any changes.

• Raise carbohydrate intake to more than half of total calories. Every gram of carbohydrate provides four calories.

• Keep protein intake to 12 to 20 percent of total calories. A gram of protein provides four calories as well.

• Lower fat intake to less than 30 percent of total calories and make every effort to substitute polyunsaturated fat or monounsaturated fat for saturated fat. Each gram of fat provides nine calories, so go easy!

• Maintain cholesterol intake at less than 300 milligrams a day. Less saturated fat in the diet will automatically lead to reduced cholesterol.

• Include fiber in the diet; it should be part of as many meals as possible.

cose levels stay normal after such sugar is ingested. "Experimenting with 'forbidden foods' may be possible with a doctor's consent," says Lebovitz. "But before you start bingeing on bonbons, it's important to be prepared to see what happens in terms of the blood-glucose response."

Get fond of fiber. The key to the effectiveness of complex carbohydrates may lie in the fiber content. "While the cause and effect of fiber in control of Type II diabetes has yet to be established, we do know that such foods are very satiating and can help enormously toward weight loss and maintenance," says Buse.

Understand "sweet" talk. Actually, there are a number of different kinds of sugar, and each has a potentially different effect on blood sugar levels. "The most basic form of sugar is glucose, or dextrose, which will raise blood sugar levels faster than any other kind when swallowed," says Ira J. Laufer, M.D., clinical associate professor of medicine at New York University School of Medicine and medical director of The New York Eye and Ear Infirmary

Diabetes Treatment Center in New York. "Sucrose also tends to raise blood sugar almost as quickly as dextrose. But fructose, sometimes called fruit sugar, generally has a very mild effect on blood sugar. If your diabetes is in good control, dietetic desserts and candies sweetened with pure fructose are not likely to raise your blood sugar levels very much," he adds. On the other hand, fructose provides as many calories as other sugars, so it may not be the wisest choice for diabetics who need to lose weight.

Reduce your risks. To emphasize the fact that excess weight is a Type II diabetic's most serious problem, experts on diabetes are fond of saying that if you want to find out if there's a possibility of getting diabetes, just keep on eating and get fat. You can do other things, too, but the main thing is get fat. An estimated 80 percent of those with Type II diabetes are obese when diagnosed with the disease. Added weight can both accelerate the diabetes and bring on its complications, especially cardiovascular disease and stroke.

In contrast, even a modest weight loss can have dramatic effects: High insulin levels drop, the liver begins to secrete less glucose into the blood, and peripheral muscle tissues begin to respond to insulin and take up glucose better. Just as obesity leads to insulin resistance, so weight loss reverses the condition. When persons with Type II diabetes lose weight, they frequently are no longer diabetic. "Type II diabetics may only need to get and stay at an ideal body weight," says Buse. "And unless they do that, nothing else will work very well." (See "Changing Your Ways" for weight-loss tips.)

Don't "crash." Too rapid weight loss rarely works in the long run and is potentially dangerous if undertaken without a doctor's advice. Sometimes, a doctor will, in fact, prescribe a very-low-calorie diet to initiate weight loss, but only for a very short period of time. Generally, the best approach is to lose weight gradually with a low-fat, lower-calorie, nutritionally balanced diet combined with increased activity. Avoid the use of over-the-counter appetite suppressants that contain phenylpropanolamine (PPA).

CHANGING YOUR WAYS

As any dieter knows, losing weight takes more "won't" power than willpower, says John Buse, M.D., Ph.D. Sometimes, people just make it too easy for themselves to fail. Here are some tips to help you succeed:

Learn what triggers your eating. If the sight of a bakery window sets off a craving for cake, make it a habit to walk on the other side of the street. Become aware of any cues like this, and learn to control them.

Don't keep large amounts of food on hand. For some overweight people, the fact that food is within reach means that it must be eaten. Buy only enough for a few meals at a time.

Prepare your meals from scratch rather than relying on take-out. For one thing, take-out foods are likely to be high in calories because of the methods used in preparation. And you might easily order too much and thereby overeat.

Graze. Many experts believe that a Type II diabetic may more easily achieve normal blood sugar levels by not overloading with too much food at one time. "Three smaller meals a day—breakfast, lunch, and dinner—plus two or three snack-type meals in between is easier for the diabetic person's insulin to handle. Just be sure that you don't overshoot your calorie limit, however," advises Lebovitz.

Get a firm foothold. Neuropathy, damage to the nerves, is a common problem for diabetics. It occurs most often in the feet and legs, and its signs include repeated burning, pain, or numbness. "Neuropathy can be dangerous if it causes a loss of feeling, because then even a minor foot injury may go undiscovered—leading to serious infection, gangrene, and even amputation of the limb," says Joseph C. D'Amico, D.P.M., a podiatrist in private practice in New York. Diabetics need to be diligent about foot care. (See "Foot Notes for Diabetics" on page 88.)

Be a sport. Regular exercise provides many benefits. It tones up the heart and other muscles, strengthens bones, lowers blood pressure, strengthens the respiratory system, helps raise HDL (good cholesterol), gives a sense of well-

FOOT NOTES FOR DIABETICS

A common complaint from many people is, "My feet are killing me!" For a diabetic, the statement could be all too true. Loss of nerve function, especially on the soles of the feet, can reduce feeling and mask a sore or injury on the foot that, if left unattended, can turn into an ulcer or gangrene. "A person with diabetes must be super cautious about foot care," says Joseph C. D'Amico, D.P.M. "Remember, there's only one pair per person per lifetime."

Here's how to start at the bottom:

Look them over. Give your feet a thorough going-over every night to make sure that you haven't developed a sore, blister, cut, scrape, or any other tiny problem that could blow up into big trouble. If your vision isn't good, have someone with good eyesight check your feet for you.

Wash, rinse, and dry thoroughly. A clean foot is a healthy foot, with a much lower susceptibility to infection. And clean feet feel better, too.

Avoid bathroom surgery. Under normal circumstances, there is little danger from using a pumice stone to reduce a corn or callus. But for a diabetic, such a practice might lead to a little irritation, then a sore, then infection, and finally, a major ulcer.

Remove "removers" from reach. Caustic agents for removing corns and calluses can easily cause a serious chemical burn on a diabetic's skin. Never use them.

Take care of the little things. Any time a cut, sore, burn, scratch, or other minor injury appears on a diabetic's foot, it must be attended to immediately. "Wash the lesion with soap and water to remove all foreign matter. Cover with a protective sterile dressing. Use adhesive tape with caution, if at all, because it can weaken the skin when it is pulled off. Use paper or cloth-type tape instead," suggests D'Amico. If the sore is not healing or if you notice signs of infection, such as redness, red streaks, warmth, swelling, pain, or drainage, see a podiatrist.

Choose shoes with care. "Since a person with diabetes may not always be aware of the pain caused by shoes that are too tight, he or she must be very attentive to fit when buying new shoes," says D'Amico.

being, decreases tension, aids in weight control, enhances work capacity, and confers a sense of achievement. "For those with diabetes," says Laufer, "exercise bestows additional benefits. It promotes the movement of sugar from the bloodstream into cells, where it is burned for energy, and it improves the cells' ability to respond to insulin, thus decreasing their need for the hormone."

Not all exercises are for every diabetic person. If blood sugar is high, exercise will lower it; if it's low, exercise will lower it further. Those on medication must work with a doctor to make necessary adjustments. Because of the potential for neuropathy, diabetics need to protect the nerve endings in the feet and so may need to avoid high-impact activities such as jogging. Another consideration is that diabetics are particularly sensitive to dehydration. Also, intense exercise could endanger capillaries in the eyes already weakened by diabetes, leading to rupture, vision problems, and even blindness. So you will need to choose your exercise program carefully with the aid of your doctor. And, especially if you are over 40 years old, you will need to undergo a general medical examination, including a cardiovascular screening test and exercise test, before proceeding with your exercise program.

Once your doctor gives you the go-ahead to begin a program of regular exercise, you need to set up realistic goals in order to avoid too-high or too-low blood sugar levels and other problems that could result from doing too much too soon. "Someone who has not spent much time engaged in physical activity who is also overweight should not be thinking in terms of running races," advises Laufer.

Swimming, bicycle riding, and brisk walking are all recommended. Indeed, walking is the one activity that all medical experts agree is ideal for a diabetic patient. "The average Type II diabetic patient is over 50, overweight, and underactive," says Laufer. Walking is a kinder, gentler activity for such individuals. Remember, however, that the positive effects of exercise last for only a day or two, so your goal should be to exercise at least every other day.

Watch your mouth. Diabetics must be extra careful about their teeth. "Good dental hygiene is important for everyone," says Andrew Baron, D.D.S., a dentist and clinical associate professor at Lenox Hill Hospital in New York. "Because they are at increased risk for infection, diabetics should be super cautious about preventing tooth decay and periodontal disease." Keep a supply of toothbrushes so you won't have to deal with old, worn brushing aids. Brush and floss without fail after every meal and before bedtime. And see your dentist regularly for checkups and cleaning.

Check your dentures. Ill-fitting dentures or permanent bridgework cause frustration for anyone who has to live with them. For a diabetic, the consequences go far beyond annoyance. "Dentures that move around in your mouth can cause sores that don't heal," cautions Baron. "It's a shame to suffer with such problems, especially when they are so easily remedied by a dentist." If you notice sore spots in your mouth or find that your dentures are moving or slipping, see your dentist to have the problem corrected.

Take charge. How do you psych yourself up for a game that has no timeouts and that never ends? That's the question diabetics face every day. One way is to learn all you can about your illness so that you can better control it. "Diabetics are constantly learning and relearning lifestyle changes and behavior adjustments. It's like studying for a master's degree in diabetes—and, in this case, there is no graduation and no vacation," says Laufer.

It's a given that even in a diabetic whose disease appears to be totally under control, there will be occasional rapid and even violent swings in blood sugar levels, brought on by emotional or physical stresses, meals, medications, or even the time of day. But if they are anticipated and accepted, these episodes can be viewed as simply a bump in the road rather than a major detour.

Do something nice for yourself. While it's important to learn as much as you can about your diabetes and stay with your treatment regimen, you also need to keep things in perspective. "It is a rare individual who takes time to 'stop and smell the roses,' as it were," notes Laufer. "This is especially true for diabetics, who often get so caught up in their disease that it is difficult for

them to focus on other, more-positive aspects of life."
Make a list of all the things you would like to do if you
had the time—and then make the time to do at least
some of them. Obviously, finishing a box of chocolates
should not appear on this list. While staring into space
may be an ideal uplifter for one person, and napping the
afternoon away does the same for another, straightening out a messy closet may do the trick for a third.

Do something nice for someone else. It's hard to think of
your own problems when you are engaged in making
another person's life more pleasant. In any city or town
in the country, there are those who are less well-off, with
more-severe problems. "You can call your local hospital
or library to inquire about volunteers," says Laufer. "Or
you can knock on the door of an elderly, housebound
neighbor who might appreciate a visit."

DIARRHEA

14 Ways to Go with the Flow

You may blame it on a 24-hour bug or something you ate,
but if you're like the average American, you'll suffer once
or twice this year from diarrhea—frequent, watery bowel movements that may be accompanied by painful cramps or nausea and vomiting.

Gastroenteritis—the catch-all medical term for intestinal
flu, viral infection, and food poisoning—is the second leading cause of missed work time (the common cold beats it).

Diarrhea is uncomfortable and unpleasant, but generally
no big deal in otherwise healthy adults. However, if diarrhea
becomes a chronic condition, the situation changes. If it affects the very young, the elderly, or the chronically ill, it can
be dangerous. And if you're not careful to drink enough fluids,
you could find yourself in trouble.

What causes diarrhea? Because the condition generally lasts
only a few days, doctors don't usually culture the stool to di-
agnose what started it in the first place. It's most often due to
a viral infection, which antibiotics can't fight. You just have to

HELLO, DOCTOR?

"If you see blood in your stool, that should immediately ring a bell to see your doctor," says Rosemarie L. Fisher, M.D.

If you feel like you're getting dehydrated, get medical attention. The signs: Dizziness when you stand up, scanty and deeply yellow urine, increased thirst, dry skin. Children may cry without tears as well.

If you've got a fever or shaking chills, or the diarrhea persists past 48 to 72 hours, see the doctor.

If diarrhea occurs in the very young, the elderly (see "The Young and the Old" on pages 94 and 95), or the chronically ill, a doctor should be consulted immediately.

tough it out for a couple of days. The virus has invaded the bowel, causing it to absorb excessive fluid, which leads to the watery stools. You may also experience cramping, nausea and vomiting, headache, fever, malaise, and even upper-respiratory-tract symptoms, such as a runny nose. One clue: If members of your family all get sick, but at different times, it's likely a virus that got passed around. Bacteria, which often cause traveler's diarrhea in certain parts of the world, can also be responsible for diarrhea as the result of food poisoning. "When the whole family goes on a picnic and six hours later, they're all sick, that's a classic sign of food poisoning," says Rosemarie L. Fisher, M.D., professor of medicine in the Division of Digestive Diseases at Yale University School of Medicine in New Haven, Connecticut.

Much rarer are microbes like amoebae and giardia that try to set up permanent housekeeping in your bowel, causing diarrhea that lasts for weeks or months. You can get these from contaminated food or water, public swimming pools, and communal hot tubs.

Certain drugs, especially antibiotics, can have diarrhea as a side effect. Magnesium-containing antacids and artificial sweeteners such as sorbitol are often overlooked culprits.

Unless diarrhea persists, you usually don't find out its cause. Treatment is aimed at relieving symptoms and preventing dehydration, the most serious consequence of diarrhea. Here's what you can do:

Ride it out. If you're not very young or old or suffering from any chronic illness, it may be safe just to put up with it for a couple of days. "Although there's no definite proof that diarrhea is a cleansing action, it probably serves some purpose," explains Richard Bennett, M.D., assistant professor of medicine at Johns Hopkins University School of Medicine in Baltimore.

Keep hydrated. In the meantime, make sure you "maintain your fluid and electrolyte balance," as the doctors say. Obviously, you can lose a lot of liquid in diarrhea, but you also lose electrolytes, which are minerals like sodium and potassium, that are critical in the running of your body. Here's how to replace what you're losing:

• Drink plenty of fluids. No one agrees on which fluid is best—again, because of the electrolyte problem. The experts do agree you need at least two quarts of fluid a day, three if you're running a fever. Plain water lacks electrolytes, although you may want to drink this part of the time. Weak tea with a little sugar is a popular choice. Some vote for Gatorade, although Fisher points out it's constituted to replace fluids lost through sweating, not for diarrhea, a whole different ball game. Defizzed, nondiet soda pop is recommended by some, although anything with a lot of sugar can increase diarrhea. So can caffeine. Fruit juices, particularly apple and prune, have a laxative effect, but others may be OK.

• Buy an over-the-counter electrolyte replacement formula. Pedialyte, Rehydralyte, and Ricelyte are available over-the-counter from your local drugstore. These formulas contain fluids and minerals in the proper proportion.

Keep your liquids cool but not ice-cold. Whatever you choose to drink, keep it cool, suggests Peter A. Banks, M.D., director of Clinical Gastroenterology Service at Brigham and Women's Hospital and lecturer on medicine at Harvard Medical School, both in Boston. It will be less irritating that way. Sip, don't guzzle; it will be easier on your insides.

Sip some chicken broth. Or any broth, says Banks. But have it lukewarm, not hot, and add some salt.

THE YOUNG AND THE OLD

For most people, diarrhea is nothing more than a minor inconvenience. But for the very young and the elderly, it can be life threatening, even fatal.

Why is it so dangerous for these groups? "Young children have a much smaller blood volume," explains Harry S. Dweck, M.D., director of the Regional Neonatal Intensive Care Unit at Westchester Medical Center in Valhalla, New York. What constitutes "a small fluid loss in an adult can make a big difference in an infant."

Dehydration can take days to occur in an adult, hours to days for a child, and seconds to minutes in a newborn, Dweck emphasizes. That's why diarrhea has been such a killer of children in many countries around the world.

If your child has diarrhea, "call the doctor right away, with the first loose stool," Dweck stresses.

Diarrhea may be harder to recognize in infants. "Newborns may have up to six to nine bowel movements a day," Dweck says. "And if they're breast-fed, it's a more liquid stool." But parents generally learn fast what their baby's normal stool looks like. If it becomes more liquid, if it's explosive, or if the odor changes, it's probably diarrhea. "The best way by far to prevent diarrhea in infants is to breast-feed," Dweck points out. The colostrum, the special milk produced during the first few days of the baby's life, "is loaded with antibodies and white blood cells" that are absorbed directly into the baby's gastrointestinal tract, which will help prevent gastrointestinal infections down the road.

There's also less chance of contamination with breast-feeding, since bottles don't have to be washed. And formula itself can cause allergic reactions that include diarrhea.

Rest in bed. Give your body a chance to fight the bug that's causing this.

Put a heating pad on your belly. Banks says it will help relieve abdominal cramps.

Try yogurt. You'll want to make sure you get a product that contains live lactobacillus cultures, which are friendly bugs that normally live in the gut. "There are anecdotal reports but no good studies that yogurt works," says Bennett. "But there's no harm in trying."

Diarrhea is less serious in children over 18 months of age, but diarrhea still warrants a call to the doctor. Your physician will tell you how to treat your baby and what to give him or her to prevent dehydration and electrolyte imbalance. Once kids reach the age of eight or so, you can follow the same recommendations for treating diarrhea as you would for adults.

The elderly can't stand to lose much fluid, either, but that's because their circulatory system has changed with aging. Hardening of the arteries occurs throughout the blood vessels in the body; lowered blood pressure that occurs when fluid is lost means there's not enough pressure to force blood to circulate.

"That puts them at a high risk for stroke, heart attack, or kidney failure," explains Richard Bennett, M.D.

But when the elderly have diarrhea, it's often difficult to know when they're becoming dehydrated. "They don't recognize thirst as well," says Bennett. "Or maybe they can't get around well enough to get a drink when they are thirsty." Changes in the skin that signal dehydration also aren't apparent in aged skin. The best clue: Are they still passing urine every hour or two?

If you're older and in good health but have a history of congestive heart failure and/or are taking diuretics, you should call your physician as soon as the diarrhea starts. "The doctor may want to change your dosage of diuretics, since these drugs cause you to lose fluid," says Bennett.

Ironically, medical care can lead to some cases of diarrhea in the elderly, says Bennett. They're more likely to be on antibiotics, which can have diarrhea as a side effect. They're also prone to constipation, and may self-medicate or have a physician recommend several types of laxatives, which can end up responsible for diarrhea. About half of the cases of diarrhea in the elderly are probably due to infections, the majority of which are viral.

Eat light. Soups and gelatin may go down easy. Banks recommends bland foods like rice, noodles, and bananas. Potatoes, toast, cooked carrots, soda crackers, and skinless, defatted chicken are also easy on the digestive system.

Take the pink stuff. Stopping the diarrhea with an over-the-counter medication may not be the best thing for your body. After all, diarrhea probably reflects your body's attempt to get rid of a troublesome bug. If you do feel it's necessary, however, Pepto-Bismol is probably the safest

WHEN DIARRHEA LASTS AND LASTS AND LASTS

Sometimes diarrhea goes on . . . for weeks. That's when a more serious problem is probably responsible. Your doctor can ferret out the cause. Here are some of the possibilities:

Lactose intolerance. "If you get diarrhea every time you drink a glass of milk, you may suffer from this condition that involves an inability to digest lactose, the sugar in milk and dairy products. It's the most common reason for chronic diarrhea," says Rosemarie L. Fisher, M.D. Avoid milk, but take a calcium supplement, she suggests.

Celiac disease. In this case, you can't digest gluten, which is part of wheat.

Irritable bowel syndrome. Emotions play a big role in this one, which can include alternating constipation and diarrhea. "The classic picture is the young adult with diarrhea on the morning of a big exam," says Fisher.

Parasitic infections. As mentioned previously, these may hang on indefinitely.

Crohn's disease or ulcerative colitis. These two conditions are similar, and no one knows their cause. But the end result of these is inflammation of the bowel and diarrhea, often accompanied by pain.

Systemic illnesses. Chronic diarrhea may be a complication of diseases such as diabetes, scleroderma, and hyperthyroidism.

Cancer. It's not a pleasant thought, but one of the warning signs of tumors in the bowel is diarrhea, especially if blood is present.

over-the-counter antidiarrheal medicine you can choose, according to Bennett. And studies show that the pink stuff may have a mild antibacterial effect, which would be most useful in traveler's diarrhea, since this condition is usually bacteria related.

Take Kaopectate or Imodium A-D. Again, you're probably better off going without antidiarrheal medication. If you absolutely need some relief, however, you can try one of these over-the-counter medications. Imodium A-D slows down the motility, or movement, of the gut; Kaopectate absorbs fluid. Bennett does not recommend these for elderly patients because decreased motility can be dangerous in an infection and can lead to worse problems.

Don't do dairy. Avoid milk or other dairy products like cheese during the time that you're having diarrhea as well as for one to three weeks afterward. The small intestine, where milk is digested, is affected by diarrhea and simply won't work as well for a while. "Milk may sound soothing," says Fisher. "But it could actually make the diarrhea worse."

Cut out caffeine. Just as it stimulates your nervous system, caffeine jump-starts your intestines. And that's the last thing you need to do in diarrhea.

Say no to sweet treats. High concentrations of sugar can increase diarrhea. The sugar in fruit can do the same.

Steer clear of greasy or high-fiber foods. These are harder for your gut to handle right now. It needs foods that are kinder and gentler.

DRY HAIR

11 Tips for Taming it

Your hair feels like straw—dry, fly-away, unmanageable. How could you have been cursed with such a mane? You probably weren't, according to Frank Parker, M.D., professor and chairman of the Department of Dermatology at Oregon Health Sciences University in Portland. "While some people are born with hair that tends to be more dry, most dry hair problems aren't organic or genetic problems at all. They're instead due to what you're doing to your hair," he says.

That's right. Those dry locks are most likely your own fault. Exposing your hair to harsh chemicals such as hair dyes, permanent-wave solutions, and the chlorine in swimming pools and hot tubs dries out the hair. So does shampooing too often and using styling tools such as hot combs, hot rollers, and blow dryers. Even too much sun and wind can dry out your tresses.

DRY HAIR

You can learn to treat your dry hair with T.L.C. and teach it to be more manageable. Here's how:

Don't overdo the shampoo. Overshampooing is one of the most common causes of dry hair, according to Parker. "Too often, people think they have to shampoo their hair every day with harsh shampoos," he says. "It just strips away the natural oils."

On the other hand, you shouldn't go too long without a good lather. "Shampoo at least every three days," says barber, cosmetologist, and hair-care instructor Rose Dygart, owner of Le Rose Salon of Beauty in Lake Oswego, Oregon. "Gentle shampooing stimulates the oil glands."

Be kind to your hair. Dygart says dry hair is the most fragile type of hair and is subject to breakage, so it must be handled with care. "Learn to shampoo your hair very gently," she says. "Try not to pull the hair or put any tension on the hair shafts."

When lathering, avoid scrubbing with your fingernails, which can not only break the hair but can irritate your scalp. Work up a lather using your fingertips, instead.

Use a gentle shampoo. Dry hair needs a gentle, acidic cleanser, says Dygart. "Use a shampoo with a pH of between 4.5 and 6.7 for dry hair. Use a gentle cleanser you wouldn't be afraid to put on your face," she says. Some people recommend baby shampoos, but Dygart says their pH is far too high, and alkaline shampoos dry out the hair. Instead, she recommends acidic shampoos.

Pour on the conditioner. Dry hair needs conditioning, says Nelson Lee Novick, M.D., associate clinical professor of dermatology at Mount Sinai School of Medicine in New York. "Find a conditioner that has as little alcohol as possible in it, because alcohol is drying," he says. "Products that have little or no fragrance usually have less alcohol. For really dry hair, try an overnight conditioner that you put on and wear a shower cap over and rinse off the next day."

For severely dry, damaged hair, Novick recommends using Moisturel, a body lotion that contains petrolatum and glycerin, instead of a conditioner. Apply the moisturizer to damp hair, and leave it on overnight beneath a shower cap. Rinse it out thoroughly in the morning.

Pour the hot oil. "Hot oil treatments are excellent for restoring dry hair," says Dygart. She recommends using over-the-counter hot oil products that you heat and place on the hair for 5 to 20 minutes (according to package instructions). Wear a plastic bag or shower cap over your hair while the hot oil is on. Then, wash the hair thoroughly with a gentle shampoo.

Slather on the mayo. Mayonnaise is another excellent moisturizing treatment for dry hair, says Dygart. "Use old-fashioned mayonnaise, not diet or low-cholesterol types," she says. "First, shampoo your hair, then apply about a tablespoon of mayonnaise. Wrap the hair in a plastic bag for 20 to 30 minutes. Then shampoo and rinse thoroughly."

Nix the 100 strokes. Novick says that because dry hair is so fragile, too much brushing can actually fracture the hair, causing hair fall. He suggests brushing gently and never brushing the hair when it is wet.

Dygart says the type of hairbrush you use is important. She recommends boar-bristle brushes or "vent" brushes, ones with rubberized tips that don't pull the hair excessively.

Give yourself a scalp massage. One way to stimulate the oil glands on the scalp is to gently massage the scalp during shampoos, says Dygart. "Use the tips of your fingers to very gently massage all over your scalp," she says. "It not only stimulates the oil glands, it also feels great."

Be an egghead. Dygart suggests beating an egg in a cup and, with tepid water (not hot—it cooks the egg!), lathering the egg into the hair and then rinsing it out with tepid water. There's no need to shampoo afterward. The egg not only cleans the hair but gives it a lovely shine.

Pace your hair treatments. If you perm on Tuesday, dye your hair on Thursday, and put it in hot rollers on Saturday, your hair is destined to be dry and damaged. "Think about your hair like a sweater," says Novick. "How many times can you dye it repeatedly before it begins to look terrible?" Novick says people with dry hair don't necessarily have to abandon styling practices like dyes, permanent waves, or hair straightening, but he says it's important to space those treatments out.

Hold the heat. Using hot combs, hot rollers, and blow dryers is asking for dry hair trouble, says Paul Contorer, M.D., chief of dermatology for Kaiser Permanente in Beaverton, Oregon, and clinical professor of dermatology at Oregon Health Sciences University in Portland. Hot rollers are the worst because they stretch the hair while the heat shrinks it. Hot combs also tend to stretch the hair and expose hair to heat for long periods of time.

If you must use artificial heat on your hair, Dygart suggests that you use a blow dryer on a low setting and avoid pulling or stretching the hair while drying.

DRY SKIN

16 Ways to Fight Moisture Loss

Everyone occasionally suffers from dry skin, according to dermatologist James Shaw, M.D., chief of the Division of Dermatology at Good Samaritan Hospital and Medical Center and associate clinical professor of medicine at Oregon Health Sciences University, both in Portland. "Dry skin is largely influenced by genetics and by climate and other drying factors like taking hot showers," he says.

When there's not enough water in the skin's top layer (called the stratum corneum), the skin becomes flaky, itchy, and unsightly. In extreme cases, this layer can become rough, cracked, and scaly, and chronic dermatitis (skin irritation) can develop.

Normally, the outer layer of the skin is kept moist by fluid from the sweat glands and from underlying tissues. Oil, produced by the sebaceous glands in the skin, helps to seal in that fluid. But lots of things rob moisture from the skin's outer layer. Some people simply have an outer skin layer that doesn't hold water well. Others may have less-active sweat glands. Age is also a factor in dry skin. The older you get, the less oil the sebaceous glands produce, and the drier your skin is likely to be.

One of the greatest skin-moisture robbers is low humidity. Cold, dry air, common in many areas during the winter months, sucks water from the skin. Add the drying effects of sun and/or high altitude to low humidity, and the parching is compounded. Heated or air-conditioned air in your home or office may also be dry and cause your skin to lose moisture.

Water can actually take moisture from your skin. Overbathing or bathing in hot water for long periods of time causes a repeated wetting and drying of the tissue that holds the outer layer of skin together and, over time, can make it less able to hold and retain water. "People who bathe several times a day or take lots of hot tubs are actually leaching important proteins from their skin that normally keep the skin moist," explains Frank Parker, M.D., professor and chairman of the Department of Dermatology at Oregon Health Sciences University in Portland.

Harsh soaps, detergents, household cleansers, and chemical solvents can also take their toll on the skin. These products can damage the skin's outer layer. People who must frequently wash and dry their hands often complain of red, chapped hands, so-called "dishpan hands."

While you can't keep skin away from all of the external moisture robbers, here are some tips to keep your skin moist and youthful-looking for years to come:

Moisturize, moisturize, moisturize. Always keep a lotion or cream on your skin, especially if you tend toward dry skin, says Parker. "Apply moisturizer right after you bathe, while you're still damp," he says. Pat, don't rub, yourself dry-damp with a soft towel. Apply moisturizers throughout the day whenever your skin feels dry and before retiring to bed.

Which moisturizers should you use? "The more oil a product has in it, the more protection it offers, and the thicker the product, the more it seals in moisture," says Shaw. "Thin lotions are mostly water. Cold creams are thicker and have more oil and less water. And products like Vaseline [petrolatum] are all oil."

Dermatologist Margaret Robertson, M.D., a staff physician at St. Vincent Hospital and Medical Center in

SUN AND YOUR DRY SKIN

If you're a sun worshipper who is always "working on your tan," you're also drying out your skin and increasing your risk of developing wrinkles, age spots, and skin cancer (melanoma), warns Frank Parker, M.D. "Just as the sun dries wet clothes hanging on a clothesline, it dries out the outer layer of the skin," he says. "Over time, the damage the sun does to the skin causes it to wrinkle and develop pigmentation spots."

Even more sobering is the increased risk of developing skin cancer from excessive sun exposure. People who are fair-skinned are at greater risk of developing such cancers than are darker-skinned individuals. To avoid the dry skin, wrinkles, and increased cancer risk from sun exposure, Parker suggests these tips:

Wear sunscreen. Sunscreens are rated by their sun protection factor, or SPF. The higher the SPF number, the greater the sun protection.

Cover up. Wear a lightweight, long-sleeved shirt and a hat when you're in the sun.

Avoid the sun between 10:00 A.M. and 3:00 P.M. This is the time of day when the sun's burning rays are at their strongest, so try to plan outdoor activities for earlier or later in the day.

Use lotions. If you must sunbathe, apply cream-type lotions and occasionally "spritz" your skin with mineral water to keep it moist. Keep your tanning sessions as short as possible, and moisturize afterwards.

Portland, Oregon, advises using a thick, unscented moisturizer that doesn't automatically disappear on the skin. She says you can mix water with petrolatum to form a cream that provides good moisture protection.

Take short, cool showers and baths. Hot water actually draws out oil, the skin's natural barrier to moisture loss, and can make itching worse, says Shaw. Bathe or shower only as often as really necessary and no more than once a day. If you insist on long, hot soaks, always apply a moisturizer immediately after bathing.

Use soap sparingly. Shaw advises decreasing soap and water washing. "People wash too much," he says. "Overwashing with soap and water harms the skin's outer layer."

People who suffer from chronically dry skin should take brief baths or showers and lather up only the groin, armpits, and bottoms of the feet, says Robertson. When you use soap, opt for milder, oilated or superfatted soaps such as Dove, Basis, or Aveenobar. For super-dry skin, you may have to use a soap substitute to cleanse your skin.

Don't be abrasive. Scrubbing your skin with washcloths, loofah sponges, or other scrubbing products dries your skin out even more, says Robertson. "Often, when people have dry skin, they develop scale and try to scrub it off with washcloths or sponges," she says. "But they're doing more harm than good."

Oil that bath. "Bath oils can help," says Shaw. But, he warns, if you put the bath oil in the water before you get in and get wet, the oil can coat your skin and prevent it from becoming saturated with water. Instead, he recommends adding the oil to the bath after you've been in the water for a while or applying it directly to your wet skin after bathing. (If you do add the oil to your bathwater, be sure to use extra care when getting in or out of the tub, since the oil will make the tub slippery.)

Robertson says that mineral oil makes an excellent bath oil. However, she warns not to soak, even in an oil bath, for longer than 20 minutes.

Raise the humidity. The higher the humidity, the less dry the skin. "In the tropics, where the humidity is around 90 percent, no one suffers from dry skin," says Shaw. He says once the temperature drops below 50 degrees Fahrenheit, the humidity tends to drop off too.

Sixty percent humidity is perfect for the skin. It's the point at which the skin and the air are in perfect balance and moisture isn't being drawn from the skin into the air. If you live in a dry climate or if the humidity in your office or home is less than 60 percent, consider using a home humidifier. Even a vaporizer or kettle of water on slow boil can raise the humidity in a room somewhat.

Avoid detergents, cleansers, and solvents. Common household products, such as cleansers, window cleaners, ammonia, turpentine, lighter fluid, and mineral spirits can dry and damage the skin's outer layer. Avoid directly exposing your skin to such products by wearing vinyl gloves and using less-harsh alternatives (for example, vinegar and water make a great window cleaner) whenever possible. Use a long-handled brush to keep your hands out of dishwater.

Nix alcohol-based products. Some people like to cleanse their faces with alcohol wipes or astringents. They leave the skin feeling clean and tingling, but there's a price. "Alcohol-based products have a drying effect," says Shaw.

Use cream- or oil-based makeup. If you wear foundation and blusher, choose oil-based types that help retain moisture rather than water-based products, says Robertson. In the evening, wash off makeup with mild soap. Then, rinse thoroughly, blot dry with a soft towel, and moisturize well with a heavy, cream-type moisturizer.

Cool it off. Hot environments heated by wood stoves or forced air heating systems dry out the skin. Shaw recommends keeping the air temperature a few degrees lower to keep your skin moist.

Toss off the electric blanket, pile on the comforter. The heat from electric blankets can dry out your skin, too. Shaw says that for people who have chronically dry skin, opting for an extra blanket instead of an electric one is a good idea.

Avoid too much alcohol. The effects of excessive alcohol consumption usually don't show up on the skin for several years. "We don't really know if there's a cause-and-effect relationship between drinking alcohol and dry skin," says Robertson. "But we do know that alcoholics tend to have drier, more wrinkled skin."

Each time you drink alcohol, your skin loses moisture needed to keep it young-looking. When alcohol enters the bloodstream, it lowers the water concentration of the blood. To replace the lost water, the body draws water from surrounding cells. Limit your intake to no more than two ounces per day. Better yet, avoid alcohol altogether.

FEVER

7 Ways to Manage the Ups and Downs

You're drenched in sweat. Your head is filled with a dull, throbbing ache, and, worse, you feel like someone is pressing their thumbs against your eyelids. One minute you feel afire; the next minute you are overcome with shaking chills. You put a thermometer under your tongue, and the mercury climbs to 101 degrees Fahrenheit. Yep, you have a fever.

To understand what having a fever means, and what you should or shouldn't do about it, it helps to know something about how the body controls temperature. There is quite a range in what is considered normal in body temperature. (By the way, *everyone* has a *temperature;* when it rises above what is considered normal and stays there, it is termed a *fever*.) The body's natural temperature-control system, located in a tiny structure at the base of the brain called the hypothalamus, is normally set somewhere around 98.6 degrees Fahrenheit. A normal temperature measured orally ranges from 96.7 to 99.0 degrees Fahrenheit (taken rectally, it measures one degree Fahrenheit higher). Your own temperature probably varies by more than two degrees during the course of a day, with the lowest reading usually occurring in the early morning and the highest in the evening.

Fever is not a disease in itself but a symptom of some other condition, usually an infection caused by bacteria, fungi, a virus, or parasites or even an allergic reaction. When this enemy invades, white blood cells are triggered to attack, releasing a protein called endogenous pyrogen. When endogenous pyrogen reaches the brain, it signals the hypothalamus to set itself at a higher point; if that new set point is over 100 degrees Fahrenheit, you have a fever.

Here's some advice on what to do when that happens:

Let it be. The fact is, fever may do the body some good. An untreated fever tends to be self limited, relatively benign, and—contrary to popular belief—not likely to escalate to the point that it causes harm. Nor does lowering a fever mean that you are lessening the severity of the illness; indeed, fever may be the body's way of mobilizing itself against invading organisms. "Over more than a decade of research, studies show that elevated body temperatures can enhance the immune response," says Matthew J. Kluger, Ph.D., professor of physiology at the University of Michigan Medical School in Ann Arbor. This heightened immune response is brought about by pyrogen, the same protein that causes the hypothalamus to reset itself. And pyrogen also has the ability to withhold iron from the blood, which apparently keeps infectious organisms from feasting and flourishing. "By leaving a fever untreated, you may be following Mother Nature's way of dealing with infection," says Kluger. There are, however, some noteworthy exceptions to this "let it be" approach (see "Hello, Doctor?" for more information on when to call the doctor). In addition, if you are feeling truly miserable, there are some steps you can try to make yourself more comfortable when you have a fever.

Dress comfortably. Let your body tell you what to wear during the course of the fever. If, as the fever is developing, you get the chills, bundle up until you feel more comfortable. On the other hand, if you feel uncomfortably warm, shed some clothing. With your body exposed as much as possible, your sweat glands will be better able to release moisture, which will make you feel more comfortable. "The fewer the clothes, the faster the fever will go down," says Pascal James Imperato, M.D., professor and chairman of the Department of Preventive Medicine and Community Health at State University of New York Health Science Center at Brooklyn. Avoid overbundling an infant.

Don't go under cover. Unless you have the chills, bundling yourself in bed under a pile of blankets or quilts will only hold the heat in and make you more uncomfortable. "Forget everything you've heard about 'sweating the fever out' by piling on the covers," advises Harold Neu, M.D., professor of medicine and pharmacology at Columbia University College of Physicians and Surgeons in New York. Once again, let your body be your guide. If a light sheet makes you feel more comfortable, don't feel that you have to bury yourself under blankets.

HELLO, DOCTOR?

Letting a fever run its course is not the best idea for everyone. While a fever of 102 to 103 degrees Fahrenheit is not usually dangerous in an otherwise healthy adult, it can be risky for very young children, who can develop seizures, and very elderly individuals, in whom fever can aggravate an underlying illness, such as a heart arrhythmia or respiratory ailment. Infants, young children, and very elderly individuals should be monitored carefully, and a physician should be called if the temperature continues to rise. Even in otherwise healthy adults, if a high fever (above 102 degrees Fahrenheit) lasts for more than a couple of days, a doctor should be consulted. Keep in mind, too, that if you or your child has a fever or other symptom that worries you, it never hurts to contact your doctor for advice.

Dip. If you feel uncomfortably warm, sponge yourself with tepid water or sit in a tub of shallow, tepid water and splash the water over your body. Don't fill the tub with water, since it's the evaporation of the water from the skin that helps cool you down. "Make sure the water is not ice cold, which can be counterproductive, since it will cause shaking and make the fever rise again. Avoid alcohol altogether because it can be absorbed into the skin and cause intoxication and dehydration," advises Imperato.

Sip. Fever, especially if it is accompanied by vomiting or diarrhea, can lead to fluid loss and an electrolyte imbalance. "Keep yourself well hydrated," says Neu. Cool water is best, but unsweetened juices are OK if that's what tastes good. Getting a child to drink plenty of water is sometimes difficult; try Popsicles or flavored ices, which are primarily water.

Don't force food down. "Don't force yourself to eat if you don't feel like it when you have a fever," says Imperato. Your body will tell you when it's time to eat. Be sure, however, to keep up your fluid intake.

Take two aspirin. Drugs known as antipyretics seek out the pyrogen and put it out of commission. Aspirin and acetaminophen are both antipyretics. However, "do not give

HOW TO READ A FEVER

"**F**eeling your forehead doesn't even give a good guess about your body temperature," says Harold Neu, M.D. "You must use a fever thermometer to get an accurate reading."

There are two basic types of glass fever thermometers, oral and rectal, with the only difference being in the shape of the bulb: thin and long on the oral and short and stubby on the rectal. Rectal temperatures are the most accurate; oral temperatures can be thrown off by breathing through the mouth, smoking, or having just had a drink of something hot or cold. Rectal readings are, in general, one degree Fahrenheit higher than oral temperatures. (If neither of these methods is convenient, temperature can also be taken by placing an oral thermometer under the armpit for at least two minutes, which will give a reading about one degree Fahrenheit lower than an oral temperature.)

Glass thermometers have several disadvantages: They may break in handling or even in the mouth. If a thermometer breaks in the mouth, don't worry; there is only a tiny amount of mercury in the tube. Just be sure to remove any slivers of glass from the mouth. Glass thermometers also need to be shaken down to 96 degrees Fahrenheit in order to allow the body's true temperature to register. On the other hand, glass thermometers have a big advantage: They are inexpensive, with most selling for about three dollars.

More convenient—and somewhat more expensive (costing about seven to ten dollars)—are newer digital thermometers, which register temperatures accurately within a tenth of a degree. These thermometers are also fast. It takes less than a minute for the temperature to register as compared to three minutes with glass thermometers. Most digital thermometers run on a "button" (or hearing-aid type) battery that boasts a two- to three-year life under normal use.

Pharmacies generally carry a selection of both glass and digital thermometers.

aspirin to a child who has or is suspected to have chicken pox, influenza, or even a minor respiratory illness," warns Imperato. "This may trigger a potentially fatal condition known as Reye's syndrome," he adds. Stick with acetaminophen for children, and follow package directions carefully.

FLATULENCE

11 Ways to Combat Gas

For stand-up comedians, the subject of flatulence is sure to generate lots of snickering, giggles, and guffaws. But for those who suffer from this distressing—not to mention embarrassing—problem, it's no laughing matter.

Everyone passes a certain amount of flatus—or "breaks wind," as we delicately describe it. Normally, from 400 to 2,000 milliliters of oxygen, nitrogen, carbon dioxide, hydrogen, and methane are expelled each day from the anus. Most of the time, this happens without inviting notice through sound or smell. But under some circumstances and in some people, undigested food products pass from the small intestine into the large intestine (colon), where the mass is fermented by large amounts of bacteria that are normally present there. The benign bugs of the colon are not choosy. Whatever comes their way goes right on their menu. It is the bacterially produced gas that gives flatus its characteristic odor when expelled.

If you are a stoic or a recluse, you may simply be able to ignore that gaseous excess and its audible effects. If you're neither, there are some things you can do to prevent or relieve flatulence. Here's how:

Eat to beat it. "Carbohydrates may be problematic for some people," says Lawrence S. Friedman, M.D., associate professor of medicine at Jefferson Medical College in Philadelphia. But before you cut out nutritious carbohydrates, try eliminating simple carbohydrates—those refined sugars, like fructose and sucrose, and white-flour foods that may taste good but are not very good for you, especially if you have a flatulence problem.

Minimize milk consumption. "Milk—the so-called perfect food—does cause gas for some people," says Sharon Fleming, Ph.D., associate professor of food science in the Department of Nutritional Sciences at the University of California at Berkeley. Some people don't have enough of the enzyme lactase in their gut or intestine to digest the milk sugar lactose. Drinking skim milk and buttermilk instead won't solve the problem either; the lactose is in the nonfat part. Cultured buttermilk may have a little less lactose, but the taste doesn't agree with everyone. If you cut down on or eliminate milk for a few days and you still have a flatulence problem, however, you can feel assured that milk is not the cause.

Add a little enzyme. If you are lactose intolerant but don't want to give up milk, you can try one of the over-the-counter products, such as Lactaid and Dairy Ease, that contain lactase enzyme, which helps to break down lactose. Be sure to follow the package directions carefully.

Banish the offenders. "Some foods are known to be flatulogenics—or flatus producers," says Norton Rosensweig, M.D., associate clinical professor of medicine at Columbia University College of Physicians and Surgeons in New York. He recommends giving up the most common ones (see "Gassers" for a list of these) and then when you feel that the flatulence problem has been relieved, start adding the foods back one by one. If your body can tolerate small quantities, you can gradually increase your intake of them.

Soak your beans. Beans are a great source of fiber and protein, but for many people, eating them can be an "explosive" enterprise. Rather than give up beans, however, you can try adjusting the way you prepare them. Mindy Hermann, R.D., a registered dietitian and spokesperson for the American Dietetic Association, suggests the following technique for decreasing the flatulogenic effects of beans: Soak the beans overnight, then dump the water out. Pour new water in, and cook the beans for about half an hour. Throw that water out, put in new water, and cook for another 30 minutes. Drain the water out for the last time, put new water in, and finish cooking.

Try Beano. This over-the-counter food modifier contains an enzyme that breaks down some of the sugars that can cause gassiness. You may find that it helps make foods such as beans, cabbage, broccoli, carrots, oats, and other vegetables and legumes more tolerable. Follow the package directions.

GASSERS

"People who suffer with chronic flatulence may be able to control the problem by eliminating foods that increase fermentation activity, thereby producing gas," says Norton Rosensweig, M.D. Here are some possible culprits:

Extremely flatulogenic:

Beans	Broccoli	Carbonated	Milk (for lactose
Beer (dark)	Brussels sprouts	beverages	intolerant)
Bran	Cabbage	Cauliflower	Onions

Mildly flatulogenic:

Apples (raw)	Carrots	Eggplant	Radishes
Apricots	Celery	Lettuce	Raisins
Bananas	Citrus fruits	Potatoes	Soybeans
Bread and	Coffee	Pretzels	Spinach
other wheat	Cucumbers	Prunes	
products			

Stay calm, cool, and collected. Emotional stress can play a major role in worsening a flatulence problem. The gastrointestinal tract is exquisitely sensitive to emotions such as anxiety, anger, and depression. A network of nerves connects this area of the body to the brain, and when you are under stress, muscles in the abdomen tighten. The results are painful spasms. "Eating while under stress also makes you swallow air, which can worsen the problem," says Friedman.

Get physical. Sometimes, flatulence is less a matter of a faulty diet than of a faulty digestive process; the smooth passage of foods down the digestive tract may be hindered in some way. Exercise helps to regulate the process, notes Friedman, who recommends taking a walk when things get uncomfortable. You can also apply pressure to your abdomen or lie facedown on the floor with a pillow bunched up under your abdomen to help relieve discomfort. Lying on your back and rocking back and forth on the floor with your knees drawn up to your chest and your arms wrapped around your legs may also help. So might a heating pad set on warm and placed on your abdomen.

Bust the belch. Excessive belching can also cause problems with flatulence.

Get activated. Activated charcoal tablets, available without a prescription, may help to absorb some excess gas and calm flatulence. If you are taking any prescription medications, however, ask your pharmacist whether the activated charcoal will interfere with them.

Reach for relief. A variety of nonprescription preparations containing simethicone (such as Mylanta and Maalox) may ease gassiness.

FLU

6 Ways to Cope with the Flu-Bug Blahs

Yesterday, you felt fantastic. Today, you feel 100 years old and counting. Your head aches, your skin feels sore to the touch, and you're chilled to the bone even though your forehead is on fire. Welcome to the wonderful world of the flu virus.

"People use the term 'flu' to describe any viral, upper-respiratory-tract infection. But strictly speaking, influenza is a very distinctive viral agent," says Marcia Kielhofner, M.D., a clinical assistant professor of medicine at Baylor College of Medicine in Houston, Texas. "Flu viruses occur yearly and attack almost exclusively between the months of October and April," she continues.

As far as who gets the flu, it seems to occur initially in children. "We'll start to see an increasing level of absenteeism within the schools and an increasing number of children hospitalized for some sort of respiratory illness. Following that, we'll see adults being hospitalized with pneumonia or with worsening of an underlying heart or lung problem," she explains.

While there are two major strains of the flu virus—influenza A and influenza B—each strain changes slightly from year to

HELLO, DOCTOR?

Signs that it's time to see your doctor include a high fever that lasts more than three days, a cough that persists or gets worse (especially if associated with severe chest pain or shortness of breath), or a general inability to recover. These things could signal a secondary bacterial infection that would need to be treated with prescription antibiotics. Marcia Kielhofner, M.D., also urges individuals with underlying lung or heart disease to consult their physician at the first sign of the flu.

year, so being infected one year doesn't guarantee protection against the flu the following year. "Every once in a while, we'll get what's referred to as a 'pandemic.' This is when we see an entirely new type of influenza virus that is associated with a much higher rate of infection and death. The last one reported in the United States was in 1977," says Kielhofner.

Regardless of the strain, the symptoms are generally the same. They include a high fever, sore throat, dry cough, severe muscle aches and pains, fatigue, and loss of appetite. Some people even experience pain and stiffness in the joints. Usually, the aches, pains, and fever last only three to five days. The fatigue and cough, however, can hang on for several weeks.

The change in flu strains from year to year also makes it hard to develop 100 percent effective flu vaccines. "We tend to make vaccines that contain antibodies to the previous year's strain, which presents a real obstacle to fully protecting people from the flu each year," explains W. Paul Glezen, M.D., a pediatrician in the Influenza Research Center, a professor of microbiology and immunology and of pediatrics, and chief epidemiologist at Baylor College of Medicine in Houston. Still, flu vaccines are about 80 percent effective when received before the flu season begins (ideally in September or October). So, if you really can't afford to get sick, a flu shot may not be a bad idea. If you fall in a high-risk group (see "Should You Get a Flu Shot?" on page 114), a flu shot is a priority.

On the other hand, if you don't manage to outrun this relentless bug, you can do a few things to ease some of the discomforts and give your body a chance to fight back.

SHOULD YOU GET A FLU SHOT?

Anyone who wants to reduce their chance of getting the flu should consider being vaccinated against the flu. However, it is especially important for the following groups of individuals to get a flu shot, according to Evan T. Bell, M.D., and Marcia Kielhofner, M.D.:

• Individuals with chronic heart and lung disease. The flu virus can aggravate these conditions to the point of causing serious complications and even death.

• People over the age of 65, especially if living in a nursing home or chronic-care facility. Viruses spread more rapidly in such environments. What's more, the flu virus attacks the already weakened immune systems of elderly people, which can lead to pneumonia and even death.

• People with other chronic diseases, such as asthma, diabetes, kidney disease, or cancer. Any time the body is fighting one disease, getting another illness can cause serious problems.

• Children who take aspirin regularly for problems such as chronic arthritis. Again, Reye's syndrome may be triggered by the flu virus in children who are on aspirin therapy.

• Health-care providers. While catching the flu may not seriously endanger these individuals, it can be deadly to the patients they are treating.

• Pregnant women who fall into any of the high-risk groups mentioned. The vaccine must be given after the first trimester of the pregnancy to prevent the possibility of harming the fetus.

Get plenty of rest. "This is especially important due to the high fever that accompanies the flu," says Evan T. Bell, M.D., a specialist in infectious diseases at Lenox Hill Hospital in New York. This shouldn't be hard to do considering fatigue is one of the main symptoms. You won't feel like doing much other than lounging in bed or on the couch. Consider it a good excuse to take a needed break from the daily stresses of life. And if you absolutely must continue to work, at least get to bed earlier than usual and try to go into the office a little later in the morning.

Take aspirin, acetaminophen, or ibuprofen—if you must. "One of the characteristic symptoms of influenza is a high fever that ranges anywhere from 102 to 106 degrees

Fahrenheit," says Kielhofner. "Headaches are also seen almost universally with influenza," she adds. Lowering the fever will help to prevent dehydration and will cut down on the severe, shaking chills associated with fever. On the other hand, since a fever may actually help your body fight the influenza bug (see "Influenza Myths"on page 116), you may want to try to let the fever run its course if you can. "The aspirin- and ibuprofen-containing drugs tend to work better against the aches and pains, while the acetaminophen works best on the fever," says Bell. But both doctors warn that people who have a history of gastrointestinal problems and/or ulcer disease should avoid taking aspirin and ibuprofen, because these medications have been shown to further complicate these conditions. And Glezen adds that individuals aged 21 and under should avoid taking aspirin during the flu season because the combination of aspirin and the flu in this age group has been associated with Reye's syndrome, an often-fatal illness characterized by sudden, severe deterioration of brain and liver function.

Drink, drink, drink. This doesn't mean alcoholic beverages, of course. But drinking plenty of any other nonalcoholic, decaffeinated liquid (caffeine acts as a diuretic, which means that it actually increases the loss of fluid from the body) will help to keep you hydrated and will also keep any mucous secretions you have more liquid. "Clear broth that is salty and warm tends to agree with people when they have the flu and are experiencing a general loss of appetite," says Glezen. Juices are also good for keeping some nutrients coming in when you're probably not eating much else.

Humidify your home in winter. "Influenza viruses survive better when the humidity is low, which explains why they tend to show up more during the winter, when we use artificial heat to warm our homes," says Glezen. Humidifying your home in the winter not only helps to prevent the spread of flu, it also makes you feel better once you have it. "When you are really sick, a little extra humidity in the form of a warm- or cool-mist humidifier works wonders," he adds.

INFLUENZA MYTHS

Despite evidence to the contrary, there are a few myths about the flu that continue to prevail. One myth has to do with what people often refer to as the "24-hour flu." This is an illness characterized by the sudden onset of vomiting and diarrhea, accompanied by a general feeling of malaise. It can be quite intense in the first few hours but tends to subside completely after 24 hours. While this illness is indeed caused by a viral agent, it is not caused by the influenza virus, and so therefore is not a form of the flu at all, according to Evan T. Bell, M.D. The correct term for this type of upset is "gastroenteritis," which indicates an infection of the gastrointestinal tract.

Another common myth about influenza is that being cold or chilled makes us more susceptible to it (as well as to the common cold). According to W. Paul Glezen, M.D., several scientific studies on humans have shown that those exposed to severe temperatures for several hours fare no worse as far as becoming ill than those who are kept warm and dry. The myth is perpetuated because severe chills are one of the first symptoms of the flu, leading people to believe that they somehow "caught a chill" that led to the illness.

An additional myth is the belief that using medicine to keep the fever down helps us to get over the illness. "Experimental studies on the flu in animals show that more of the virus is excreted over a longer period of time when the body temperature is lowered with medication," says Glezen. "So while such treatments may make you feel better, they don't necessarily help you get over the virus."

Suppress a dry cough. For a dry, hacking cough that's keeping you from getting the rest you need, you can reach for over-the-counter relief. "Cough remedies containing dextromethorphan are best for a dry cough," says Kielhofner.

Encourage a "productive" cough. A cough that brings up mucus, on the other hand, is considered productive and should not be suppressed with cough medicines. Drinking fluids will help bring the mucus of a productive cough up and will ease the cough a little as well, according to Glezen.

HEADACHES

16 Ways to Keep the Pain at Bay

Headaches. We've all had them. From the morning-after-celebrating-too-much headache to the tough-day-at-the-office headache to the you-might-as-well-kill-me-now-because-I'm-going-to-die-anyway headache. Sometimes, an aspirin or other analgesic may ease the pain; at other times, nothing short of waiting it out seems to help.

If you suffer from frequent, severe headaches that put you out of commission several times a month, you need to seek medical attention. Likewise, if your headaches are associated with physical exertion, changes in vision, or weakness, numbness, or paralysis of the limbs, skip the urge to self-treat and see a doctor. If you're already seeing a physician and aren't getting relief, think about getting a referral to a headache specialist or headache clinic.

However, if you are prone to occasional headache pain, read on. The tips that follow can help you feel a lot better—fast.

Don't overdo the pain pills. Although an occasional dose of an over-the-counter analgesic may help alleviate your headache for a few hours, taking these drugs too often may actually worsen the pain, according to Sabiha Ali, M.D., a neurologist at the Houston Headache Clinic in Texas. "These drugs are OK in limited quantities," she says, "but if you need to take more than two doses a day, you should see a doctor."

Lie down. Lying down and closing your eyes for half an hour or more may be one of the best treatments for a bad headache. For some types of headaches, such as migraines, sleep is the only thing that seems to interrupt the pain cycle. "The most important thing is to recognize that the faster the patient with a severe headache stops what they're doing and goes to bed and rests, the faster the headache will go away," says James R. Couch, Jr., M.D., Ph.D., professor and chairman of the Department of Neurology at the University of Oklahoma Health Sciences Center in Oklahoma City. "You need to recognize when the big headache is coming. That's the time to give up and go to bed."

HEADACHE RESOURCES

The following associations provide support and information for headache sufferers:

The American Council for Headache Education (ACHE). ACHE provides patient information and referrals to headache specialists. The organization also sends out free informational pamphlets about headache treatment. In the future, ACHE plans to set up patient-support groups around the country. You can contact ACHE at 1-800-255-ACHE.

The National Headache Foundation. This organization sends out free headache information to patients and publishes a headache newsletter. You can contact the Foundation at 1-800-843-2256.

Don't let the sun shine in. Especially if the symptoms that you are experiencing resemble those of a migraine headache (such as severe pain on one side of the head, nausea, blurred vision, and extreme sensitivity to light), resting in a darkened room may alleviate the pain. Bright light may also cause headaches, according to Seymour Diamond, M.D., founder of Diamond Headache Clinic in Chicago. "Sometimes, looking at a computer screen may bring on a headache," he says. "Tinted glasses may help."

Use a cold compress. A washcloth dipped in ice-cold water and placed over the eyes or an ice pack placed on the site of the pain are other good ways of relieving a headache, says Fred D. Sheftell, M.D., director and founder of The New England Center for Headache in Stamford, Connecticut. (A bag of frozen peas or frozen unpopped popcorn works well as an ice pack.)"Other good solutions are the 'headache hat,' which is an ice pack that surrounds the head, and the ice pillow, which is a frozen gel pack that is inserted into a special pillow," he says. (These special ice packs can be found in some pharmacies; if you don't see them at yours, ask your pharmacist about ordering them.) Using ice as soon as possible after the onset of the headache will relieve the pain within 20 minutes for most people, Sheftell adds.

Try heat. If ice feels uncomfortable to you, or if it doesn't help your headache, try placing a warm washcloth over your eyes or on the site of the pain, Ali says. She recommends leaving the compress on for half an hour, rewarming it as necessary.

Think pleasant thoughts. Many headaches are brought on or worsened by stress and tension, according to Couch. Learning to handle life's difficulties in a calm way may keep the volume down on a bad headache, he says. "Turn off all thoughts of unpleasant, crisis-provoking things," he says. "Think about pleasant things. Just for the moment, try to forget about the confrontation with the boss or the coworker. Try to relax while you work out a strategy to cope with the problem."

Check for tension. Along with the preceding tip, Sheftell recommends that patients periodically check their body for tension throughout the day. "If you notice that you get these headaches frequently, check the body for signs of tension," he says. "Are your jaws set very tightly? Are you scrunching your forehead? You want to check to see if your fists are clenched. Also, when you stop at a red light, are your hands gripping the wheel very tightly?" If the answer to any of the questions is yes—stop, relax, and take a deep breath or two (don't go beyond a couple of deep breaths, though; otherwise, you may begin to hyperventilate).

Quit smoking. Smoking may bring on or worsen a headache, Couch says, especially if you suffer from cluster headaches—extremely painful headaches that last from 5 to 20 minutes and come in groups.

Don't drink. Alcohol, aside from its notorious morning-after effect, may also bring on migraines and cluster headaches, according to Diamond. Alcoholic beverages contain tyramine, an amino acid that may stimulate headaches (see "Dr. Diamond's Antiheadache Diet" on pages 122 and 123 for a listing of other foods that contain tyramine).

Start a program of regular exercise. Regular exercise helps to release the physical and emotional tension that may lead to headaches, according to Ali. She recommends

RECIPES FOR RELAXATION

In addition to being given an antityramine diet (see "Dr. Diamond's Antiheadache Diet" on pages 122 and 123), patients at Diamond Headache Clinic in Chicago are instructed in relaxation techniques. The following is a typical relaxation exercise. The exercise can be memorized, or the written instructions can be recorded on a cassette tape. The entire exercise, which relaxes the facial area, neck, shoulders, and upper back, takes about five minutes. Before you begin, make sure you won't be disturbed—close the door and take the phone off the hook.

1. Settle back quietly and comfortably into a favorite chair or sofa. Allow your muscles to become loose and heavy.

2. Wrinkle up your forehead, hold it, then smooth it out, picturing the entire forehead becoming smoother as the relaxation increases.

3. Frown, creasing your eyebrows tightly, feeling the tension. Let go of the tension, smoothing out your forehead once more.

4. Close your eyes more and more tightly. Feel the tension as you hold them shut. Relax your eyes until they are closed gently and comfortably.

5. Clench your jaws and teeth together. Feel the tension build, then let go and relax, letting the lips part slightly. Allow yourself to feel relief in the relaxation.

6. Press your tongue hard against the roof of your mouth. Again, feel the tension, then relax.

7. Purse your lips together more and more tightly, then relax. Notice the contrast between tension and relaxation. Feel the relaxation all over your face, forehead and scalp, eyes, jaws, lips, and tongue.

8. Press your head back against your chair, concentrating on the tension in the neck. Roll your head to the right and feel the tension shift. Repeat to the left. Straighten your head and bring it forward, pressing chin to chest. Finally, allow your head to return to a comfortable position.

9. Shrug your shoulders up to your ears, holding the tension, then drop. Repeat the shrug, then move the shoulders forward and backward, feeling the tension in your shoulders and upper back. Drop the shoulders and relax.

10. Allow the relaxation to spread deep into the shoulders, into your back. Relax your neck and throat. Relax your jaws and face. Allow the relaxation to take over and grow deeper and deeper. When you are ready, slowly open your eyes.

walking or jogging. These and other aerobic activities, she says, help to boost the body's production of endorphins (natural pain-relieving substances).

Cut down on caffeine. "Caffeine can increase muscle tension and your anxiety level," Sheftell says. "It also creates difficulties in sleeping, which can cause headaches." Another problem is that many people drink several cups of coffee a day during their work week but cut their consumption on weekends. This can lead to weekend caffeine-withdrawal headaches, according to Sheftell. "My advice to those people is for them to slowly decaffeinate themselves," he says. "Decrease your caffeine intake by one-half cup per week. I suggest that people who are prone to headaches cut down to the equivalent of one cup of caffeinated coffee per day," says Sheftell. One five-ounce cup of drip coffee contains about 150 milligrams of caffeine. A five-ounce cup of tea brewed for three to five minutes may contain 20 to 50 milligrams of caffeine. And cola drinks contain about 35 to 45 milligrams of caffeine per 12-ounce serving. Sheftell also recommends checking the caffeine content of any over-the-counter drugs in your medicine cabinet.

Fight the nausea first. Some headaches may be accompanied by nausea, which can make you feel even worse. What's more, the gastric juices produced by stomach upset may hinder the absorption of certain over-the-counter and prescription analgesics, which may make these drugs less effective at relieving the pain of your headache. So, by first taking care of the nausea, the pain of the headache may be easier to treat, says Sheftell. He says that many of his patients have found that drinking peach juice, apricot nectar, or flat cola has helped alleviate nausea. Over-the-counter antinauseants such as Emetrol and Dramamine may also be useful.

Rise and retire at the same time every day. Going to bed and getting up at the same time every day also helps prevent headaches, according to Diamond. "Changes in body chemistry that occur when you oversleep can precipitate migraines or other headaches," he says.

(Continued on page 124)

DR. DIAMOND'S ANTIHEADACHE DIET

At Diamond Headache Clinic in Chicago, patients are advised to eat a diet low in tyramine, an amino acid that is known to promote headaches, nausea, and high blood pressure in certain individuals. People who take certain antidepressant drugs called monoamine oxidase (MAO) inhibitors are especially prone to accumulating high amounts of tyramine. The following diet keeps tyramine levels to a minimum.

BEVERAGES

Foods allowed: Decaffeinated coffee, fruit juices, club soda, noncola sodas. Caffeine sources to be limited to no more than two cups per day.

Foods to avoid: Caffeine (does not contain tyramine, but aggravates headache symptoms): coffee, tea, colas in excess of two cups per day. Hot cocoa, all alcoholic beverages.

DAIRY

Foods allowed: Milk: homogenized, low-fat, or skim. Cheese: American, cottage, farmer, ricotta, cream cheese. Yogurt: limit to one-half cup per day.

Foods to avoid: Cultured dairy, such as buttermilk, sour cream, chocolate milk. Cheese: blue, boursault, brick, Brie types, Camembert types, cheddar, Swiss, Gouda, Roquefort, Stilton, mozzarella, Parmesan, provolone, Romano, Emmentaler.

MEAT, FISH, POULTRY

Foods allowed: Fresh or frozen turkey, chicken, fish, beef, lamb, veal, pork, eggs (limit three per week), tuna fish.

Foods to avoid: Aged, canned, cured, or processed meats; canned or aged ham; pickled herring; salted, dried fish; chicken liver; aged game; hot dogs; fermented sausages (no nitrates or nitrites allowed), including bologna, salami, pepperoni, summer sausage; any meat prepared with meat tenderizer, soy sauce, or yeast extracts (it's not the yeast itself that's a problem, but yeast contains an enzyme that alters an amino acid to become tyramine).

BREADS AND CEREALS

Foods allowed: Commercial breads: white, whole wheat, rye, French, Italian, English muffins, melba toast, crackers, bagels. All hot and dry cereals: cream of wheat, oatmeal, cornflakes, puffed wheat, rice, bran, etc.

Foods to avoid: Hot, fresh, homemade yeast breads; breads and crackers containing cheese; fresh yeast coffee cake, doughnuts, sourdough breads; any breads or cereals containing chocolate or nuts.

STARCHES

Foods allowed: Potatoes, sweet potatoes, rice, macaroni, spaghetti, noodles.

VEGETABLES, LEGUMES, AND SEEDS

Foods allowed: Asparagus, string beans, beets, carrots, spinach, pumpkin, tomatoes, squash, corn, zucchini, broccoli, green lettuce. All vegetables, legumes, and seeds except those listed in the next paragraph.

Foods to avoid: Pole, broad, lima, or Italian beans; lentils; snow peas; fava, navy, or pinto beans; pea pods; sauerkraut; garbanzo beans; onions (except when they are used as a condiment); olives; pickles; peanuts; sunflower seeds; sesame seeds; pumpkin seeds.

FRUIT

Foods allowed: Prunes, apples, cherries, apricots, peaches, pears. Citrus fruits and juices: Limit to one-half cup per day of orange, grapefruit, tangerine, pineapple, lemon, or lime.

Foods to avoid: Avocados, bananas (one-half allowed per day), figs, raisins, papaya, passion fruit, red plums.

SOUPS

Foods allowed: Cream soups made from list of allowed foods, homemade broths.

Foods to avoid: Canned soups, bouillon cubes, soup bases with autolyzed yeast or monosodium glutamate (MSG)—read labels.

DESSERTS

Foods allowed: All of the fruits that are listed above in the "allowed" category; sherbets; ice cream, cakes and cookies made without chocolate or yeast; gelatin.

Foods to avoid: Chocolate-flavored ice cream, pudding, cookies, or cakes; mincemeat pies.

SWEETS

Foods allowed: Sugar, jelly, jam, honey, hard candy.

Foods to avoid: Chocolate bars and other chocolate candies, chocolate syrup, carob.

MISCELLANEOUS

Foods allowed: Salt (in moderation); lemon juices; butter or margarine; cooking oils; whipped cream; white vinegar and commercial salad dressing in small amounts.

Foods to avoid: Pizza, cheese sauce, soy sauce, monosodium glutamate (MSG) in excessive amounts, yeast, yeast extracts, Brewer's yeast, meat tenderizers, seasoning salt, macaroni and cheese, beef stroganoff, cheese blintzes, lasagna, frozen dinners, and any pickled, preserved, or marinated foods.

Keep a headache diary. If you get frequent headaches, try
to tease out the factors that seem to be responsible, says
Sheftell. "Pick up patterns. Figure out a way to record
headaches and rate them on a zero-to-three scale of intensity: no headache, mild headache, moderate to severe
headache, incapacitating headache. Start to look at what
foods you are eating. Women should begin tracking their
periods, as well as their use of hormone-replacement
medications or oral contraceptives. You can show this
calendar to your doctor."

HEARTBURN

21 Ways to Beat the Burn

Heartburn. The word evokes a frightening picture: Your
heart on fire, sizzling and smoking, without a fire fighter
in sight. Fortunately, the word is a misnomer. It's not your
heart that's on fire, it's your esophagus. But heartburn is easier to say than "esophagusburn."

The "burn" part, however, they got right. Your esophagus,
the tube that carries what you swallow down to your stomach, can be burned by the acids released by your stomach.
Those acids are industrial-strength stuff and are meant to stay
where the tough stomach lining can handle them.

Unfortunately, we can experience something called reflux.
That's when some of the stomach contents, including the
acid, slip back up through the esophageal sphincter, the valve
that's supposed to prevent the stomach's contents from re-
versing course.

David M. Taylor, M.D., a gastroenterologist and assistant
professor of medicine at Emory University in Atlanta and at
the Medical College of Georgia in Augusta, puts it plainly: "If
it goes south, that's good; if it goes north, you're in trouble."

Reflux causes an uncomfortable burning sensation between
the stomach and the neck. Most people feel the discomfort
right below the breastbone.

The easy way to avoid a simple case of heartburn?
Moderation. Heartburn is generally the result of eating too

HEIMLICH MANEUVER WON'T HELP THIS

Heartburn can become very serious, says Douglas C. Walta, M.D. The acid reflux of heartburn can sometimes burn the lining of the esophagus so badly that scar tissue will build up. The resulting strictures can cause food to get stuck in the esophagus.

A person with a piece of food stuck in his or her esophagus can still breathe and talk, says Walta. "It doesn't interfere with breathing, but if it totally occludes, all of a sudden you can't swallow your saliva."

The Heimlich maneuver, used for dislodging an object that is obstructing the airway, is not the appropriate treatment in this case. Usually, a doctor must use a special instrument that is inserted into the esophagus to dislodge the food. So if it feels as if you have food stuck in your esophagus or if you are having trouble swallowing your saliva, see a doctor.

much too fast. But if it's too late for moderation, here are some things you can do to put out that fire and keep it from flaring up in the future.

Take an antacid. Over-the-counter antacids in tablet or liquid form can help cool the burn. Take a dose about every six hours as needed, says Nalin M. Patel, M.D., a gastroenterologist in private practice and clinical instructor at the University of Illinois at Urbana-Champaign. Don't overdo it, though, because too much antacid can cause constipation or diarrhea.

Don't forget your bedtime dose. Even if you forget to take an antacid during the day, try to remember to take one at bedtime to protect yourself from the pooling of stomach acids.

"Nighttime damage is probably the worst that will occur, because you're bathing your esophagus in acid, and you're much more prone to burn it," says Douglas C. Walta, M.D., a gastroenterologist in private practice in Portland, Oregon. Try keeping a bottle of antacid on your nightstand so that you remember to take your nightly dose.

IS IT REALLY HEARTBURN?

If symptoms don't subside, you may have something other than a simple case of heartburn.

"Persistent heartburn can be a sign of significant disease," warns David M. Taylor, M.D. "They [persistent-heartburn sufferers] can have hiatal hernia or esophagitis [inflammation of the esophagus], they can have an ulcer in their stomach, they can have an ulcer in the duodenum [part of the small intestine], and in an older person, they can even have cancer. And sometimes heartburn can mimic coronary disease, and they can have heart trouble."

The best advice: If symptoms persist, see your doctor.

Keep your head up. Another way to protect your esophagus while you sleep is to elevate the head of your bed. That way, you'll be sleeping on a slope, and gravity will work for you in keeping your stomach contents where they belong. Put wooden blocks or bricks under the legs at the head of your bed in order to bring it up about six inches, advises Patel.

Have a glass of milk. Milk can sometimes cut the acid and decrease heartburn, says Taylor.

Get rid of your water bed. "People with water beds who have reflux have to get rid of their water beds," says Walta. "They don't like to hear that." The problem with a water bed is that your body basically lies flat on the water-filled mattress. You can't effectively elevate your chest and so can't keep your stomach contents from heading north.

Say no to the couch. Tempting as it may look, the couch is not your friend after eating a meal. People who lie down with a full stomach are asking for trouble. "Stay upright for one hour after meals," says Patel.

Don't eat before bed. Heading from the dinner table to bed is a no-no for heartburn sufferers. In fact, doctors recommend warding off sleepy time for two to three hours after a meal. And by that, they mean staying upright for that amount of time. "You should stay upright until the gastric contents are emptied," says Walta.

Pass on seconds. "If you overeat, it's kind of like a balloon," says Walta. "If you blow it up real tense, it's more likely to empty quickly if you release the valve." A stomach ballooned by too much food and drink may partly empty in the wrong direction.

Loosen your belt. "Avoid tight clothing around the waist," says Patel. "This tends to increase acid backing up into the esophagus."

Lose the fat. If you're fat on the outside, you can be sure you're fat on the inside, too, says Walta. "The fat competes for space with your stomach." Fat pressing against the stomach can cause the contents to reflux.

Don't blame the baby. For the same reason that fat can impede normal digestion—competition for space—pregnancy can cause heartburn. That's all the more reason expectant mothers should watch what they eat and give up that nonsense about eating for two. Remember, pregnant or not, you only have one stomach. Be sure to discuss with your doctor any questions you may have about proper diet and weight gain during pregnancy.

Get in shape. "Couch potatoes have heartburn," states Taylor. "You almost never have heartburn when you exercise." Even mild exercise done on a regular basis, such as a daily walk around the neighborhood, may help ease digestive woes. However, avoid working out strenuously immediately after a meal; wait a couple of hours.

Watch your diet. "A high-carbohydrate, low-fat, high-bulk diet is the best thing," says Taylor. Fried foods and fatty foods should be avoided, he says, because they take longer to digest. Highly spiced foods sometimes contribute to heartburn as well.

Don't smoke. Nicotine from cigarette smoke irritates the valve between the stomach and the esophagus, as well as the stomach lining, so smokers tend to get more heartburn.

Be careful of coffee. It may not be the caffeine that's the problem. The oils contained in both regular and decaffeinated coffee may play a role in heartburn. Try cutting your coffee intake to see if your heartburn troubles subside.

Be wary of peppermint. For some people, peppermint seems to cause heartburn. Try skipping the after-dinner mints and see if it helps.

Hold the pepper. For people with heartburn problems, using pepper is not such a hot idea, says Kimra Warren, R.D., a registered dietitian at St. Vincent Hospital and Medical Center in Portland, Oregon. Sprinkling or grinding pepper, whether red or black, onto your food may be contributing to your heartburn troubles, so try going easy on it.

Take it easy. "A big contributor to heartburn is stress," says Taylor. Stress can create increased acid secretion and can cause the esophageal sphincter to malfunction.

Don't crack open a cold one. Alcohol can relax the sphincter, notes Taylor. It can irritate the stomach, too, which can lead to reflux.

Slow down on soda. Carbonated beverages and soda pop can contribute to heartburn woes. "Carbonation causes stomach distention due to gas, and that causes acid rolling back up into the esophagus," Patel explains.

Check your painkiller. If you're about to pop a couple of aspirin in your mouth, think again. Aspirin, ibuprofen, and products that contain them can burn the esophagus as well as the stomach, warns Walta. Opt for acetaminophen instead.

HEMORRHOIDS

14 Ways to End the Torment

When was the last time you heard a party conversation turn to the subject of hemorrhoids? The condition is rarely discussed, even between close friends and relatives, although Americans spend $150 million a year on remedies that promise relief.

Hemorrhoids are swollen and stretched-out veins that line the anal canal and lower rectum. Internal hemorrhoids may either bulge into the anal canal or protrude out through the anus, in which case they are called "prolapsed." External hemorrhoids occur under the surface of the skin at the anal opening. Regardless of type, hemorrhoids cause cruel distress: They hurt, burn, itch, irritate the anal area, and, very often, bleed.

About one-half to three-fourths of all Americans will develop hemorrhoids at some time in their lives. The following factors contribute to them, and some can be avoided.

• Gravity. Humans stand upright, which causes a downward pressure on all veins in the body, including those in the anal canal and rectum.

• Genes. If one parent has hemorrhoids, it is more likely that his or her child will develop them in adult life; if both parents have hemorrhoids, it is an almost certain outcome.

• Age. While hemorrhoids usually begin to develop when an individual is twenty years old or even earlier, symptoms usually do not appear until the thirties and beyond.

• Constipation. Difficulty in passing fecal matter creates pressure and possible injury to veins in the anal canal and rectum.

• Low-fiber diet. Highly refined foods (white flour products, sugar, foods high in fat and protein and low in complex carbohydrate) result in a fiber-deficient diet, with resulting constipation and hemorrhoids.

• Obesity. Added pounds put more pressure on veins. What's more, overweight individuals may be more likely to favor refined foods and a sedentary lifestyle.

• Laxatives. Improper use of these products is a major cause of constipation and, as such, it may also be considered a prime factor in the development of hemorrhoids.

• Pregnancy. As the fetus grows, it puts additional pressure on the rectal area. Pregnancy-related hemorrhoids usually retract after the baby is born, unless they were present beforehand.

• Sexual practices. Anal intercourse also puts pressure on veins in the anal canal.

• Prolonged sitting. Without some form of exercise, the heart muscle works more slowly in returning blood in the body's veins to the heart.

• Prolonged standing. The pull of gravity continues unabated on the body's veins in individuals who are on their feet all day.

COULD IT BE SOMETHING ELSE?

"**O**ften people attribute symptoms to hemorrhoids when other conditions are to blame," notes Norton Rosensweig, M.D. Itching may be the result of poor anal hygiene, perianal warts, intestinal worms, medication allergies, psoriasis, other forms of dermatitis or local infection, or too much coffee. Pain can result from fissures—small cracks in the skin around the anus.

Erroneously attributing bleeding to hemorrhoids can be a serious mistake. Bleeding can be a symptom of colorectal cancer, which kills 60,000 people every year. "Rectal bleeding must be followed up promptly," cautions Rosensweig. While bright-red bleeding usually heralds hemorrhoids, don't try to make a diagnosis yourself. If you notice blood, see your doctor.

Fortunately, most cases of hemorrhoids respond to basic self-care methods, so you may never have to tell a soul about them. (If you notice blood, however, see "Could It Be Something Else?") The following are the most effective steps that you can take to soothe your achy bottom and keep hemorrhoids from flaring.

Rough up your diet. "People who consume large amounts of food containing fiber—or what grandmothers used to call 'roughage'— rarely have problems with hemorrhoids," says Thomas J. Stahl, M.D., assistant professor of general surgery at Georgetown University Medical Center in Washington, D.C. Fiber passes through the human digestive tract untouched by digestive enzymes. As it travels, it has the capacity to absorb many times its weight in water; by the time it reaches the colon in combination with digestive waste, it produces a stool that is bulky, heavy, and soft—all factors that make it easier to eliminate. "Straining to have a bowel movement day after day because of constipation is probably the main cause of hemorrhoids," says Norton Rosensweig, M.D., associate clinical professor of medicine at Columbia University College of Physicians and Surgeons in New York. According to medical experts, adding fiber to the diet is the only treatment necessary for about half of all hemorrhoid cases (see "An Apple a Day" for a listing of fiber-rich foods).

AN APPLE A DAY

One of the most important moves toward healing hemorrhoids is a change in diet. "By all means, increase your intake of fiber-rich foods—but do it gradually," advises Norton Rosensweig, M.D. Too rapid an increase can cause gas, abdominal cramps, or diarrhea. As it is, you can expect some increase in intestinal gas at first, but this will subside in a week or two as your system and the bacteria that inhabit your colon adjust.

Here are some foods that can increase the fiber content of your diet when eaten regularly:

Vegetables

Carrots	Brussels sprouts	Eggplant
Cabbage	Corn	Green beans
Lettuce		

Fruits

Apples	Pears	Figs
Prunes	Apricots	Raisins
Oranges		

Grains

Wheat, whole	Rye, whole	Rice, brown
Corn, milled	Oatmeal, unprocessed	Oats, rolled
Bran, unprocessed miller's		

Legumes

Lima beans	Soybeans	Kidney beans
Lentils	Chick peas	

Drink up. Be sure to drink lots of water to keep the digestive process moving right along. A minimum of eight large glasses of water or other fluid a day is recommended, according to Gayle Randall, M.D., assistant professor of medicine in the Department of Medicine at the University of California Los Angeles School of Medicine. And remember that fruits and vegetables, which are important sources of dietary fiber, come naturally packaged in their own water.

Avoid sweat and strain. Don't try to move your bowels unless you feel the urge to do so. And don't spend any more time on the toilet than it takes to defecate without straining. "You should not try to catch up on yesterday's read-

THOSE OVER-THE-COUNTER "SHRINKS"

Drugstore remedies for hemorrhoidal discomfort usually achieve part of what they promise: temporary relief of pain and itching. Claims that they can shrink hemorrhoids or reduce inflamed tissue, however, don't hold up when put to the test, say the experts.

Over-the-counter aids are available in three forms: cleansers, suppositories, and creams and ointments. The cleansers, although effective, are more costly than ordinary warm water, which works very well. Suppositories may be of little use, according to some experts, because they may slip up into the upper rectum, bypassing the area they are meant to soothe. Ointments are greasy and tend to retain moisture, which can lead to increased irritation. Creams, especially hydrocortisone creams, are effective; however, their prolonged use may lead to dependency and can also cause thinning of the skin.

Furthermore, while some drugstore remedies may feel good, they may cause more harm than good in the long run. Some of these products should not be used by individuals with certain medical conditions, such as heart disease or diabetes, so you'll need to check the label of any product you are considering. In addition, many preparations contain a number of ingredients, including anesthetics, astringents, counterirritants, and skin protectants, which may cause an allergic reaction in some persons that is far worse than the discomfort of the hemorrhoids themselves.

The Food and Drug Administration has also made some specific rulings about products marketed for hemorrhoidal use.

• Boric acid is no longer allowed. While it's safe enough for ordinary skin, it is toxic if absorbed by the mucous membranes.

• Painkilling ingredients are out, too, because rectal nerves don't sense pain, so such ingredients are unnecessary.

• Lanolin alcohols, cod liver oil, and Peruvian balsam are banned as ineffective rather than unsafe.

• Product labels must say "If your condition worsens or does not improve in seven days, consult your doctor."

• Product labels claiming to shrink tissue must also caution: "Do not use this product if you have heart disease, high blood pressure, thyroid disease, diabetes, or difficulty in urinating due to an enlarged prostate gland unless directed by a doctor."

Keep in mind that, according to the experts, using petroleum jelly or zinc oxide ointment or powder may be as beneficial as any "hemorrhoid preparation" you can buy.

ing while sitting on the toilet," advises Rosensweig. Once your bowels have moved, don't strain to produce more.

Heed the call of nature. On the other hand, don't wait too long before responding to the urge to eliminate. The longer the stool stays in the lower portion of the digestive tract, the more chance there is for moisture to be lost, making the stool hard and dry. "The frenzied pace many people follow today can lead to elimination always getting low priority," says Stahl.

Try a different position. It has been suggested that squatting is a more natural position than sitting for moving one's bowels; unfortunately, Western toilets are not designed to make this possible for most people. "Try putting your feet on a small footstool to raise your knees closer to your chest," advises Randall.

Soften it. Sometimes, eating more fiber-packed food and increasing water intake aren't enough to solve a severe constipation problem. In this case, you might want to ask your doctor to recommend a laxative known as a stool softener (such as Colace or Correctol) or one that contains a natural bulking agent (such as Metamucil and Effer-Syllium). Experts agree, however, that the safest and best way to add fiber to the diet is through foods. Don't—repeat don't—use laxatives that act on the muscles of the colon and rectum; prolonged use of these products can cause permanent malfunction of the bowel in addition to severe irritation of the anal area. Avoid mineral oil, as well, since it can interfere with the absorption of some essential nutrients such as vitamin A. "Ordinary laxatives are short-term solutions that lead to long-term problems," says Rosensweig.

Take a walk. Regular exercise helps your digestive system work more efficiently. No need for strenuous aerobics, however; a lengthy walk at a brisk pace will do.

Keep it clean. Keep your rectal area clean at all times. Residual fecal matter can irritate the skin, but so can vigorous rubbing with dry toilet paper. Randall's suggested solution: "Gently rinse the area with plain water while sitting on the toilet. Then pat the area dry and dust with powder, preferably nontalc and unperfumed." More convenient, but also more expensive, are premoistened wipes designed for anal care. These wipes, however, may cause irritation in some people, says Randall. If you want to try them, they are available without a prescription at pharmacies and drugstores.

Rinse well. Soap residue can also irritate the anal area. "Be sure to rinse the anal area completely after a bath or shower," says Randall.

Skip the soap. If you find that, even with thorough rinsing, soap still irritates the anal area, look for a special perianal cleansing lotion in your drugstore. Follow the package directions.

Soften your seat. If your job demands that you sit all day, try sitting on a donut-shaped cushion—an inexpensive device that takes the pressure off the sensitive area. "But it's still important to get up and walk around whenever possible," says Stahl.

Sitz around. Sit in six inches of warm water on your donut cushion or a towel twisted into a circle big enough to support your bottom. "Taken three or four times daily, a half-hour sitz bath will soothe inflamed tissues and relax muscle spasms," says Randall.

Take the heat. Even if you can't manage a full-scale sitz bath, applying a washcloth moistened with warm water can soothe the painful area.

Slim down. If you are overweight, you'll be doing your bottom a favor by getting your weight closer to the desirable range. You'll be doing the rest of your body good, too.

HIGH BLOOD CHOLESTEROL

21 Heart-Healthy Ways to Lower It

Heart attacks are the leading cause of death in the United States. In 1989 alone, says the American Heart Association (AHA), heart attacks claimed the lives of 497,850 American men and women.

What causes a heart attack? In most cases, an attack occurs when the blood supply to part of the heart muscle is severely reduced or stopped, according to the AHA. This stoppage is caused when one of the arteries that supply blood to the heart is obstructed, usually by the fatty plaques that characterize atherosclerosis, a result of coronary-artery disease.

Although it's not clear where the plaques come from in each individual case, the most common causes are a blood cholesterol level that's too high, a hereditary tendency to develop atherosclerosis, and increasing age (55 percent of all heart attack victims are 65 or older, 45 percent are under 65 years of age, and 5 percent are under 40). Other factors that contribute to the likelihood that heart disease will develop are cigarette smoking, high blood pressure, and male sex (although after menopause, a woman's risk rises to almost equal that of a man), according to the AHA.

You can't change your age, your gender, or your genes, but you can make positive lifestyle changes that can sharply reduce your risk of developing heart disease. Getting your blood cholesterol down to a level that's considered low risk (see "Low, Borderline, High—What Do the Numbers Mean?" on page 136) is an important first step. The following tips are designed to help you take that step.

Adopt a new lifestyle. Making a commitment to lowering blood cholesterol and improving your heart health requires a change of mind-set, not a temporary fad diet, according to Henry Blackburn, M.D., Mayo Professor of Public Health and a professor of medicine at the University of Minnesota in Minneapolis. "You need to adopt a healthy lifestyle, a familywide lifestyle," he says. "Even if one member of your family has a low risk of developing heart disease, that doesn't mean his or her risk will stay low. Our risk rises as we get older, and it takes a lifetime to establish good habits." Lifetime good habits also mean avoiding "yo-yo" dieting—losing weight and gaining it back repeatedly. Yo-yo dieting has been shown to cause cholesterol levels to rise.

Know it's never too early to act. Although much of the emphasis on heart disease risk is placed on people with a total blood cholesterol level over 240, the numbers can be a bit misleading, says William P. Castelli, M.D., director

LOW, BORDERLINE, HIGH—WHAT DO THE NUMBERS MEAN?

According to the American Heart Association (AHA), total levels of blood cholesterol under 200 milligrams per deciliter represent a low risk for coronary heart disease. Levels between 200 and 240 are considered to be borderline risk, and over 240 is considered dangerously high risk.

While total levels of blood cholesterol are considered important, other factors come into play, as well. For example, if someone has a borderline-high total cholesterol level, but has very low levels of HDL, the "good" cholesterol, he or she may still have a high risk of heart disease. In general, doctors worry about the ratio of LDL (the "bad" cholesterol) to HDL.

A desirable HDL level is over 50, according to W. Virgil Brown, M.D. For LDL, a level below 130 is desirable, 130 to 160 is borderline high, and over 160 represents a high risk of heart disease, he says. Although these numbers aren't absolute (for example, levels of triglycerides, another fatty acid, also enter into the big picture), they do represent a fairly good predictor of heart disease risk, according to Brown. "We know that, on average, for every one percent increase in total blood cholesterol, there is a two to three percent increase in heart disease rates," he says. "For a person with a total cholesterol of 220, their risk is ten percent higher than a person with a total cholesterol of 200. A person with a level of 250 has a 50 percent higher risk than the person with 200."

of the Framingham Heart Study in Massachusetts, the oldest and largest heart disease study in the United States. "Most heart attacks occur in people with a total cholesterol level between 150 and 250," he says. "Many doctors don't understand that. That group up at the top, the highest-risk group (with cholesterol levels above 240), only produces about 20 percent of the heart attacks." Even if you're in a low or borderline group, you still need to pay attention to your lifestyle habits, he advises.

Ignore the magic bullets. This week it's rice bran, last week it was oat bran and fish oil. All were touted as the solution to your cholesterol problem. While it's the American way to search for shortcuts, such an approach just doesn't cut it when you're dealing with your health, according to Basil M. Rifkind, M.D., F.C.R.P., chief of the Lipid Metabolism and Atherogenesis Branch at the National Heart, Lung, and Blood Institute in Bethesda, Maryland. "We are very cautionary about these magic-bullet remedies," he says. "If someone's cholesterol is high, we know that it comes about by eating a bunch of foods that are higher than the optimum in fat and cholesterol. We need to address the source of the problem, instead of paying attention to garlic, fiber, or fish oil."

Stay away from saturated fats. Many people make the mistake of believing that if their blood cholesterol level is high that it's because they ate too many foods containing cholesterol. Not exactly true, says W. Virgil Brown, M.D., past president of the AHA and professor of medicine and director of the Division of Arteriosclerosis and Lipid Metabolism at Emory University School of Medicine in Atlanta. The number-one cause of high serum cholesterol is eating too much saturated fat, the kind of fat that is found in full-fat dairy products and animal fat, he says. Another culprit is partially hydrogenated vegetable oil, which contains *trans* fatty acids, substances that increase the cholesterol-raising properties of a fat. The best rule of thumb is to stick with fats that are as liquid as possible at room temperature, according to Brown. "For example," he says, "if you are going to use margarine, use the most-liquid kinds, such as the tubs or squeeze bottles."

Read your meat. The small orange labels stuck to packages of meat at the grocery store aren't advertisements or promotions; they're actually grades of meat, says Castelli. "Prime," "Choice," and "Select" are official U.S. Department of Agriculture shorthand for "fatty," "less fatty," and "lean," he explains. "Prime is about 40 percent to 45 percent fat by weight, Choice is from 30 percent to 40 percent fat, and Select, or diet lean, is from 15 percent to 20 percent fat," he says. You could have a hamburger made from Select ground beef for breakfast, lunch, and dinner and still not exceed your daily saturated fat limit, he adds.

Learn to count grams of fat. The AHA's dietary guidelines outline the percentages of daily calories that should come from fat (see "The American Heart Association Diet"). However, since most package labels show grams of fat, not percentages, it can be difficult to figure out exactly what you're eating, Castelli says. Instead, he recommends counting grams of fat. How many grams of fat, and how many grams of saturated fat, can you have each day? Multiply your total number of calories per day by .30, then divide by 9 to find the number of grams of total fat allowed. (You divide by 9 because each gram of fat provides 9 calories.) Multiply your total number of calories per day by .10 and divide by 9 to find the number of grams of saturated fat allowed each day.

"If you're on a 2,000-calorie-per-day diet, you should eat no more than 22 grams of saturated fat a day," Castelli says. "The average American eats twice as much."

What can you eat for 22 grams of fat? One serving of Choice beef contains from 12 to 15 grams of fat, whereas a serving of Select contains 4 to 10. One tablespoon of butter is just under seven grams, while many brands of low-fat margarine contain only one gram per tablespoon. Whole milk has a whopping five grams per cup; skim milk just one. You add it up. After all, if you choose the lower-fat versions of each item, maybe you'll have enough saturated fat calories left in your daily budget to indulge in some low-fat frozen yogurt, a cup of which may contain as little as two grams of saturated fat.

Go to the extreme. Although the AHA recommends deriving 30 percent or fewer of your daily calories from fat, some heart specialists believe it's not only safer, but better, to go even lower. (The average American derives about 37 to 40 percent of his or her calories from fat.) "It's quite appropriate for a person with a high degree of risk for heart disease to go to these sort of extremes," says Blackburn. "That means reducing fats way down. You can go down even to five percent of your calories from fat without hurting yourself. We've examined populations in Japan who consume 9 percent to 12 percent of their calories from fat and they are perfectly healthy and have very low cholesterol. It's worth the effort."

THE AMERICAN HEART ASSOCIATION DIET

The following are the dietary guidelines put forth by the American Heart Association. They are designed to prevent heart attacks, stroke, and other manifestations of cardiovascular disease from occurring in healthy adults.

1. Total fat intake should be less than 30 percent of daily calories.

2. Saturated fat intake should be less than ten percent of daily calories.

3. Polyunsaturated fat intake should not exceed ten percent of daily calories.

4. Dietary cholesterol intake should not exceed 300 milligrams per day.

5. Carbohydrate intake should constitute 50 percent or more of daily calories, with an emphasis on complex carbohydrates.

6. Protein intake should provide the remainder of the calories.

7. Sodium intake should not exceed three grams (3,000 milligrams) per day.

8. Alcohol consumption should not exceed one to two ounces of ethanol per day. Two ounces of 100-proof whisky, 8 ounces of wine, and 24 ounces of beer each contain 1 ounce of ethanol.

9. Total calories should be sufficient to maintain the individual's recommended body weight, as defined by the Metropolitan Tables of Height and Weight (Metropolitan Life Insurance Company, New York, 1959).

10. A wide variety of foods should be consumed.

Eat as much like a vegetarian as possible. Dietary cholesterol is found only in animal products; animal products also tend to be higher in fat (skim-milk products are exceptions), especially saturated fat. Foods derived from plant sources, on the other hand, contain no cholesterol and tend to be lower in fat. The fats they do contain tend to be polyunsaturated and monounsaturated, which are healthier than the saturated kind, says Peter F. Cohn, M.D., chief of cardiology at the State University of New York at Stony Brook. (The exceptions are coconut oil, palm oil, palm kernel oil, and partially hydrogenated oils, which contain higher amounts of saturated fatty acids.) You'll be doing your arteries a favor if you increase your intake of vegetable proteins, such as beans, whole grains, and tofu, and keep servings of high-fat animal products to a minimum.

Increase your carbohydrate intake. Adding extra servings of complex carbohydrates into your diet will fill you up and make you feel more satisfied, leaving less room for fatty meats and desserts, says Cohn. Complex carbohydrates include fruits, vegetables, pasta, whole grains, and rice.

Grill it. Grilling, broiling, and steaming are heart-smart ways to cook food, says Brown. Unlike frying, they require no added fat.

Skin a (dead) chicken. The skin of chicken (and turkey, too, for that matter), is an absolute no-no for people who are watching their fat intake, according to Cohn. The skin contains high amounts of saturated fat, he says.

Skip the pastry. One hidden source of saturated fat is pastry—donuts, Danishes, piecrust, éclairs, and so on, says Brown. These confections are often made with shortening or butter—two things that should be limited by people who are working to reduce their saturated fat intake. Stick with whole-grain bread and rolls, and read labels to be sure you know what's in the package, he suggests.

Eat fish. Fish oil, as a cholesterol reducer, has gotten a lot of play in the media in the past few years. And it is true that the slimy stuff contains high levels of omega-3 fatty acids, substances that have been associated with lower cholesterol levels, according to Blackburn. However, the greatest benefit has been achieved in people who frequently substitute fish for their intake of higher-fat meats. Also, fish oil itself tends to be high in fat, Blackburn says. His advice is to add more servings of fish into the diet (as substitutes for some of the meat dishes) and reap the oil's benefits naturally.

Go easy on yolks. You can have all the eggs you like, as long as you leave the yolks behind. Egg yolks are more than 50 percent fat and also contain high amounts of cholesterol. Egg yolks may also be hidden inside processed foods, so be sure to read labels carefully. The AHA recommends

HEART-SMART GLOSSARY

The following are definitions of terms commonly used in discussions of cholesterol and cardiovascular health:

LDL: Low-density lipoprotein, the "bad" cholesterol often implicated in the development of atherosclerosis

HDL: High-density lipoprotein, the "good" cholesterol thought to protect against atherosclerosis

Triglycerides: Another type of fatty acid found in the blood that doctors measure when they evaluate heart-disease risk

limiting egg yolks to no more than three per week, including those found in processed foods or those used in cooking.

Eat smaller meat portions. One way to cut down on saturated fat without giving up steaks is to keep your portions small, says Brown. "Reduce the size of the meat portions, even chicken, to about three ounces per serving," he advises. "Try to have a vegetarian lunch. Then you can have six ounces at dinner." A three-ounce serving is about the size of a deck of cards, Brown says.

Give up organ meats. Like eggs, organ meats are something best left behind as a memory of foods gone by, says Brown. Although rich in iron and protein, these meats are also tremendously high in fat and cholesterol. And remember—pâté is made from liver, so it, too, should be restricted.

Increase your fiber intake. Soluble fiber, the kind found in fruits and brans, has been shown to be effective in lowering cholesterol levels, says Brown. However, to exert this effect, it must be consumed in high amounts; a bowl of oatmeal a day probably won't make much difference. "You have to eat about a quarter pound of oatmeal per day to get ten grams of soluble fiber a day, the amount that can lower cholesterol," he says. He recommends a daily one-teaspoon dose of a psyllium-husk powder, such as Metamucil, which provides a lot more bang for your buck. "For the person whose cholesterol is still borderline high after changing their diet, psyllium may give them another eight percent to ten percent reduction in their LDL," he says. And no need to go overboard, either. More than ten grams a day won't make much more of a difference, he says. It's also prudent to increase your fiber intake gradually to give your system time to adjust.

Eat like the rest of the world. "Four billion of the 5.3 billion people on this earth eat 15 grams of saturated fat or less each day," says Castelli. "Where do they live? Asia, Africa, and Latin America. They are the four billion people who never get atherosclerosis. We want our 250 million people to eat like those 4 billion. If we accomplished this, we could get rid of heart attacks, stroke, and other manifestations of cardiovascular disease. We could live five years longer, which isn't much. However, we wouldn't have heart attacks in our 40s, 50s, 60s, 70s, or 80s. That is the vision for America."

Quit smoking. Most of us are aware that smoking can cause lung cancer and raise the risk of heart attack, but few people know that smoking can actually affect your cholesterol levels, says Brown. "When you stop smoking, your HDL levels rise significantly," he explains. "A two-pack-a-day smoker who quits may have an eight-point rise in their HDL cholesterol."

Add exercise to your daily routine. Studies have shown that regular aerobic exercise can boost levels of HDL, says Brown. "Exercise can be very useful in reducing body weight, which can help cholesterol levels," he says. "When you engage in even modest amounts of exercise, your triglycerides come down, your LDL comes down, and your HDL goes up after several months." He recommends 30 to 45 minutes of moderate exercise, such as walking, five days per week. It is important to accelerate your heart rate and keep it up for at least 20 minutes, he says. However, he adds, it is not necessary to do your exercise all at once. Try parking your car a quarter mile from work and walk it twice a day. Take the stairs instead of the elevator. It all adds up.

Know it's never too late. Even if you've had a heart attack or have other evidence of heart disease, changing your lifestyle can still dramatically reduce your risk of a recurrence, says Rifkind. In the past, heart specialists thought that lifestyle changes couldn't make much of a difference for people who already had heart disease. They now believe differently. "We want the cholesterol to be much lower in these people than in their healthy counterparts," he says. "For these people, the target levels of total serum [blood] cholesterol are between 160 and 170."

HIGH BLOOD PRESSURE

13 Ways to Reduce It

At last count, 62,770,000 Americans had or were being treated for high blood pressure, according to the American Heart Association (AHA). That's almost one-quarter of our country's population. Every year, 31,630 of these individuals die as a direct result of the condition, the AHA says. An additional 147,470 deaths every year occur from stroke (a blood clot that travels to the brain), making it the number-one fatality related to high blood pressure. Another 2,980,000 Americans have had a stroke and lived. Many of these people are now severely disabled and unable to care for themselves.

High blood pressure, or hypertension, is defined as having blood pressure (the force that is created by the heart as it pumps blood into the arteries and through the circulatory system) equal to or higher than 160 systolic (the top number) over 95 diastolic (the bottom number), according to William P. Castelli, M.D., director of the Framingham Heart Study in Framingham, Massachusetts, the oldest and largest heart-disease study in the United States. Between 140 and 159 systolic over 90 to 94 diastolic is considered "borderline" high. Below these numbers is considered normal.

In addition to strokes, high blood pressure can cause blindness, kidney failure, and a swelling of the heart that may lead to heart failure.

Who's at risk for high blood pressure? People with a family history of the condition, blacks (they have an almost one-third greater chance of having high blood pressure compared to whites), overweight individuals, and aging individuals. Also

SYMPTOMS OF A STROKE

If you are experiencing any of the following stroke symptoms, call your doctor or an ambulance at once. Waiting too long or not recognizing the signs could mean the difference between life and death. If you experience any of these symptoms and then feel better within 24 hours, you may have had a transient ischemic attack, or TIA. A TIA is a warning sign that a full-blown stroke is on its way. Again—call your doctor at once.

• Sudden weakness or numbness of the face, arm, or leg on one side of the body

• Sudden dimness or loss of vision, particularly in only one eye

• Loss of speech, or trouble talking or understanding speech

• Sudden, severe headaches with no apparent cause

• Unexplained dizziness, unsteadiness, or sudden falls, especially along with any of the previous symptoms

(Source: "1992 Heart and Stroke Facts," by the American Heart Association.)

at risk are women who are pregnant or who are taking oral contraceptives.

The good news is that, together with your doctor, you can control hypertension. It won't be easy—you'll have to change the way you think and act. You may have to take medication for the rest of your life. You'll definitely have to cut out some bad habits and begin some new, more healthful ones. However, your efforts are likely to pay off in a longer, healthier life. Here's to your health!

Join the club. It may sound trivial, but the first step toward controlling your blood pressure is actually accepting that you've got a problem to begin with, says David B. Carmichael, M.D., medical director of the Cardiovascular Institute at Scripps Memorial Hospital in La Jolla, California. "People must accept the fact that they've got hypertension," he says. "The worst person in the world is an aggressive 40-year-old male who comes in feeling fine and is told he has hypertension and will have to monitor his blood pressure. They often just won't believe it. In fact, if I ask myself what type of patient has left my practice over the years, I would say it has been the hypertensives." Carmichael likens this type of acceptance to joining a fraternal lodge. "You've got to do certain things: go to the doctor, take your medications faithfully, modify your diet, report bizarre symptoms. You have got to join the club."

Lose weight. "At all levels of blood pressure, increased weight contributes to the degree of blood pressure elevation," says Robert A. Phillips, M.D., Ph.D., director of the Hypertension Section and associate director of the Cardiovascular Training Program in the Division of Cardiology at Mount Sinai Medical Center in New York. "Weight loss lowers blood pressure—not in everybody, but in many people. It's worth a try." Phillips explains that for each pound of excess body weight that is lost, blood pressure may drop by two points. "It's always a good thing to do, even if you are severely hypertensive," he says. "If you are mildly hypertensive, that weight loss may enable you to stay off of medication." Even a modest amount of weight loss is better than none at all, according to Castelli. "The most common problem in hypertension is borderline hypertension—between 140 and 159 systolic and 90 to 94 diastolic," says Castelli. "That level of blood pressure increases the risk of stroke three times. And yet, virtually all of those people would be cured with a ten-pound weight loss."

Invest in a home blood pressure monitor. If you have been diagnosed as hypertensive, or if your doctor wanted more blood pressure readings before making a definitive diagnosis, he or she may have prescribed you a home blood pressure monitor. At-home monitoring has several benefits—first and foremost, warning you if your pressure becomes dangerously high, so you can get medical attention early. Second, a monitor can save you money, because it will save you trips to the doctor. "This is now very common," says Carmichael. "It is also easy to do. If the patient is afraid to use the monitor [some people become panicky if they find their pressure is high], another person, such as a spouse, can do it for them. The blood pressure should be checked at close to the same time of day, under the same conditions." Carmichael says that most insurance companies will cover the purchase of such devices if prescribed by a physician.

PREGNANCY AND HYPERTENSION

I f you have been diagnosed as having high blood pressure and you become pregnant, you should see your doctor as soon as possible to discuss ways to control your condition during pregnancy.

During pregnancy, your blood volume triples, placing a great deal of additional strain upon the heart. Perhaps because of this increase in blood volume, many women who never had a problem with blood pressure become hypertensive, a condition called pregnancy-induced hypertension.

The problems of hypertension in pregnancy are twofold: First, the condition is extremely dangerous, posing a risk of stroke, preeclampsia (a condition that causes sudden weight gain, extreme water retention, blurred vision, and other symptoms), stillbirth, premature delivery, and low birth weight. Second, blood pressure may be difficult to control without medication, and many medications may pose a danger to the developing fetus.

However, several studies have shown that extra calcium has a definite blood-pressure-lowering effect in pregnant women, according to Johns Hopkins researcher John T. Repke, Ph.D. Repke's findings show that pregnant women may need to take between one-and-one-half and two times the recommended daily allowance of calcium to keep their blood pressure at safe levels. However, he cautions that pregnant women should check with their doctors before taking supplements or exceeding the recommended amount of any nutrient.

The recommended daily allowance for calcium during pregnancy is 1,200 milligrams per day, the amount contained in about eight servings of low-fat milk, yogurt, or broccoli.

Start an exercise program. Along with helping with weight loss, exercise confers additional benefits for those with high blood pressure, says Phillips. "For people who are severely hypertensive, they shouldn't exercise until their blood pressure is controlled," he says, "but people with mild hypertension can exercise aerobically for 20 to 30 minutes, three times per week, and will benefit with a reduction in blood pressure by about eight points that will last at least half a day." It's best to check with your doctor before beginning any exercise program, especially if you have been living a sedentary lifestyle. The types of exercise that are most likely to benefit your blood pressure are walking, jogging, stair-climbing, aerobic dance, swimming, bicycling, tennis, skating, skiing, or anything else that elevates your pulse and sustains the elevation for at least 20 minutes. Nonaerobic exercise, such as weight lifting, push-ups, and chin-ups, may actually be dangerous for people who have high blood pressure. These types of exercise should not be done without the explicit consent of your doctor.

Take your blood pressure medicine. The biggest danger with hypertension, Carmichael says, is that it is usually asymptomatic until its final stages, where it becomes fatal. That's why the condition is often labeled "the silent killer." Unlike people who have other chronic illnesses, such as diabetes, you'll probably feel just fine if you don't take your medicine. However, inside your body, the disease will continue to progress, damaging the arteries in your eyes, destroying your kidneys, causing your heart to swell, and so on. Another problem that can occur when you stop taking your blood pressure medicine is a rebound phenomenon, where the blood pressure rises to a higher level than it was before you started taking the medication. The moral of the story? "If you're starting and stopping your medication, you haven't joined the club," says Carmichael.

Cultivate a taste for less-salty foods. "There is no question that salt in the diet has a relationship with blood pressure," says Jeffrey A. Cutler, M.D., a hypertension specialist and chief of the Prevention and Demonstration Research Branch of the National Heart, Lung, and Blood Institute in Bethesda, Maryland. "We Americans take in far more salt than we need. We've become accustomed to the taste. However, the fact is that our taste sense is adaptable. People who lower the salt in their diets, after a period of time, have been shown to taste something as salty at a much lower level of salt than before." The average American takes in about eight to ten grams of salt a day, Cutler says. However, studies have shown that by cutting that amount down by a third, blood pressure can be significantly reduced, he says. Ideally, he says, people should cut down to six grams per day as a short-term goal and to about four-and-a-half grams per day as a long-term goal.

Read labels. So how do you know how much salt you're eating? As far as table salt goes, one teaspoon contains over two grams—almost half of the recommended daily amount. Also, says Cutler, the average American adult takes in somewhere between one-and-a-half to two extra teaspoons of salt a day without knowing it. These insidious salt sources are frozen entrées, canned vegetables, even antacid medications. To avoid this extra salt, read labels. Many labels will express the amount of sodium in milligrams (1,000 milligrams is equivalent to 1 gram). To calculate the amount of sodium chloride, or salt, multiply the amount of sodium by two-and-a-half, Cutler says.

Say no to a second round. Restriction of alcohol consumption to one drink (1.5 ounces of hard liquor, 4 ounces of wine, or 12 ounces of beer) per day does not appear to increase the risk of high blood pressure, but consuming two or three drinks per day is associated with an elevated risk of hypertension, according to Phillips.

Eat a banana. One substance (other than prescription medication) that has been proven to reduce blood pressure is potassium, says Cutler. However, it may be difficult to increase your intake of potassium enough to lower blood pressure, he adds. While supplements may help, they are not recommended without the permission of a doctor, since they may be hazardous in individuals with certain medical conditions. "The average person needs three to four servings of potassium-rich fruits and vegetables per day," he says. "It would probably benefit your blood pressure in a detectable way if you could double that number of servings. A little more may be a little better, and a lot more may be a lot better." Potassium-rich foods include bananas, raisins, currants, milk, yogurt, and orange juice.

Drink your milk. Some studies have shown that extra calcium added to the diet may have a modest effect on blood pressure, says Phillips. Although the effect may not be significant, there's certainly no harm in adding a few extra glasses of skim milk, low-fat yogurt, or leafy green vegetables to the daily diet, he says.

Add polyunsaturated oils to your diet. Most people know that by substituting polyunsaturated oils for saturated fats in their diets they can reduce their level of blood cholesterol. However, what most people don't know is that polyunsaturates can also reduce blood pressure, according to James A. Hearn, M.D., an assistant professor of medicine at the University of Alabama at Birmingham. "Switching to canola and safflower oils in cooking can cut your blood pressure by ten points," he says.

Quit smoking—now. Cigarette smoking is the number-one taboo for hypertensives, says Phillips. Not only does the nicotine in the smoke cause blood pressure to rise, but it dramatically raises your risk of stroke, he says. According to the AHA, cigarette smoking can thicken the blood and increase its propensity to clot. Blood clots in the arteries leading to the heart can cause a heart attack, while blood clots in the artery leading to the brain may cause a stroke, according to the AHA. The good news is, you get an immediate benefit by giving up the habit right now. "Two years after you quit smoking, your risk of developing coronary artery disease has dropped to the same level as someone who never smoked," Phillips says. In contrast, it can take much longer for a person's risk of lung cancer to drop to that level. Your doctor can be a great source of help to you in quitting smoking. He or she may prescribe nicotine gum or skin patches to reduce withdrawal discomfort. Your local Heart Association may also be able to provide you with resources.

Learn to relax. Many people misunderstand the term hypertension, believing it to mean a condition where the patient is overly tense. This isn't true. The term is defined solely by blood pressure levels. However, many hypertensives are the consummate "Type A" personality—aggressive, workaholic, hostile, frustrated, or angry, says Carmichael. For these people, some form of relaxation, be it prayer, yoga, biofeedback, or just resting, may be an important component of treatment, he says. "People need to recognize their personality traits and do their best to change," he says. Some chronically stressed-out individuals release a lot of adrenaline into their systems. That rush of hormone can constrict the arterioles (tiny blood vessels), causing them to go into spasm. It is difficult for the heart to push blood through constricted arterioles. The effect? Higher blood pressure, says Carmichael.

INCONTINENCE

20 Steps to Greater Security

Have you stopped taking an aerobics class because you're afraid you might have an "accident"? Do you worry when it's time to take a long car trip on highways with few roadside rest areas? Do you dread sneezing, coughing, even laughing, because you're not sure if you'll stay dry?

Rest assured, you're not alone. Help for Incontinent People (HIP), a not-for-profit organization in Union, South Carolina, estimates that at least 12 million, and perhaps as many as 20 million, people in the United States and Canada suffer with urinary incontinence, oftentimes in silence. Indeed, it's a problem that's only been recognized relatively recently in America as a treatable condition and not merely an unavoidable symptom of old age. As a matter of fact, other cultures in times past seemed to have been much more aware of the problem. The ancient Egyptians developed products for incontinence, and in Great Britain around the turn of the century, it was perfectly acceptable for a woman to hold what was called a "slipper" under her dress to relieve herself during a long church service.

The loss of bladder control is not a disease but a symptom with any of a host of causes. It can affect anyone at any age—from children to the elderly, both women and men. Women, however, are three times more likely than men to be incontinent, due in part to the physical stresses of childbearing and a decrease in estrogen after menopause. The cause of incontinence may be as minor as an infection triggered by a cold or the use of certain prescription or over-the-counter medications. Incontinence may also be the result of sagging pelvic-floor muscles. This set of muscles located at the bottom of the pelvis supports the lower internal organs and helps them maintain their shape and proper function. Childbirth and certain types of surgery, such as a hysterectomy in a woman (removal of the uterus) or a prostatectomy in a man (removal of the prostate gland), can cause these pelvic-floor muscles to become deficient. (See "Exercises for Incontinence" on page 155 for help in toning up the pelvic-floor muscles.)

Incontinence reveals itself in a number of ways, and one person can suffer from more than one form of it. Stress incontinence occurs from rigorous or spontaneous activity, like playing tennis or sneezing. Urge incontinence is marked by a sudden need to go but possibly not making it to the bathroom in time. Overflow incontinence is a full bladder that begins to dribble. And reflex incontinence is marked by an unawareness of the need to urinate (caused by an enlarged prostate gland, for example), which results in leakage. Here are ways to cope:

Keep a diary. "This is very helpful in establishing symptom patterns," says Katherine Jeter, Ed.D, E.T., executive director of HIP. By maintaining a voiding diary, or uro-log, you'll have a record of when you urinated and the circumstances causing it. The diary should include: the time of day of urination or leakage; the type and amount of fluid intake that preceded it; the amount voided in ounces (pharmacies carry measuring devices that fit right inside the toilet bowl); the amount of leakage (small, medium, or large); the activity engaged in when leakage occurred; and whether or not an urge to urinate was present. Keeping such a diary for at least four days, if not a full week, before you see a doctor can help him or her to determine what type of incontinence you have and the course of treatment. When you see a doctor, take along a list or the actual bottles of any prescription or over-the-counter medicines you have been taking, because some medications can cause incontinence.

Watch what you drink. Experts are not entirely sure why some beverages seem to irritate the bladder lining and, as a result, cause bladder leakage. But you may want to eliminate certain substances from your diet or at least decrease your intake of them to see if your urine control improves. The caffeine in coffee, for instance, may irritate the bladder, and the ingredients that give coffee its distinct aroma (also found in decaffeinated varieties) can be irritating, too. Tea, another favorite breakfast drink, is not only a diuretic, which means it pulls more water from the kidneys as it passes through, but also a bladder irritant. (HIP recommends substituting hot grain beverages, found in your grocer's coffee and tea aisle.) Citrus fruits and juices, such as grapefruit and tomato, can be a problem. Carbonated sodas may be irritating, too, according to HIP (you might be able to tolerate seltzer water, which is not as highly carbonated as sodas). And, finally, alcoholic beverages should be avoided. Your safest bet: water, perhaps with a twist of lemon for flavor (a few drops of lemon should not be enough citrus to cause or aggravate an incontinence problem).

Try these juices. Grape juice, cranberry juice, cherry juice, and apple juice are not irritating to the bladder and may, in fact, control the odor of your urine. And surprisingly, orange juice is not an irritant, because it is metabolized by the body into a more alkaline, or less acidic, fluid before it reaches the bladder, says Jeter.

Keep drinking. "Too often, people who suffer with incontinence limit their fluid intake, believing that the less they take in, the less they'll urinate. But dehydration can occur," warns Thelma Wells, Ph.D., R.N., F.A.A.N., F.R.C.N., a professor of nursing at the University of Rochester School of Nursing in Rochester, New York. Dehydration can lead to constipation, which in turn can irritate nearby nerves that will trigger the bladder to void. The result: incontinence. Instead of cutting back on how much you drink, schedule the time that you drink. Having liquids at set intervals during the day will keep your bladder from becoming too empty or too full. "The bladder becomes irritated if its fluid level is too low or too high," explains Wells. A normal bladder holds about two cups of fluid; problem bladders may hold as little as half a cup or as much as a quart and a half. If you find yourself constantly waking up in the middle of the night to go to the bathroom, you might try to taper off your fluid intake between dinner and bedtime, says Wells.

Experts suggest an average total fluid intake of six to ten 8-ounce cups a day.

Watch what you eat. Again, experts are not sure why certain foods aggravate the bladder, but you may want to try cutting back on the following foods to see if it helps: hot spices and the foods they're used in, such as curry powder and chili; tomato-based foods; sugars, such as honey and corn syrup; and chocolate.

Try a recipe for success. If you are constipated, adding fiber to your diet may relieve your constipation and, in turn, your incontinence. Here's an easy-to-make-snack recipe from HIP that may help. Combine one cup of applesauce, one cup of oat bran, and a quarter cup of prune juice. Store the mixture in your refrigerator, or freeze premeasured servings in sectioned ice-cube trays. Begin with two tablespoons every evening, followed by a six- to eight-ounce glass of water or juice (one of the acceptable varieties mentioned previously). After seven to ten days, increase this to three tablespoons. Then, at the end of the second or third week, increase your intake to four tablespoons. You should begin to see an improvement in your bowel habits in about two weeks. The extra fiber may cause increased gas or bloating, but this should decrease after a few weeks. Be sure to keep up your daily fluid intake in addition to using this fiber recipe.

Lose weight. Obesity can cause muscles to sag, including the pelvic-floor muscles, which aid in proper voiding.

Do not smoke. Here's another reason to give up the habit. Nicotine can irritate the bladder, and for heavy smokers, coughing can contribute to stress incontinence.

Buy yourself some insurance. There are numerous products on the market today that will absorb any accidents, whether urine or a bowel movement, and at the same time, protect your clothing or bedding from wetness. Specially made disposable and reusable briefs, diapers, liners, inserts, and linen protectors can add a measure of confidence. For some people, sanitary napkins or panty liners may be an acceptable alternative that provides enough protection. And a new product may be on the market soon. "Within the next year or two, urethral plugs, which can block the flow of urine during everyday activities, will be available in the United States," says Peter K. Sand, M.D., associate professor of obstetrics and gynecology at Northwestern University School of Medicine and director of the Evanston Continence Center at Evanston Hospital in Evanston, Illinois. These plugs, now in use in Europe, can be inserted by the user and later removed by means of an attached string.

Be confident on the road. External collecting devices that are specially designed for use by females or males can make traveling a little more comfortable. These on-the-go urinals, which are also convenient for bedside use, are available at medical-supply stores and pharmacies and through medical-specialty mail order.

Go before you go. Empty your bladder before you take a trip of an hour or more, whether you have the urge to urinate or not.

Then go again. After voiding, stand up and sit down again. Then lean forward, which will compress the abdomen and put pressure on the bladder, to help empty the bladder completely, suggests Wells.

Wear clothes that are easy to remove. Women's clothing, in particular, can pose a problem. Jumpsuits or unitards can slow you down when you're in a hurry to go because these one-piece outfits must be removed from the top down. Skip such suits or look for ones with a snapped opening at the crotch for quick-and-easy removal. Carry extra clothing with you so that you can change if an accident occurs. If your clothes happen to become stained with urine, soak them for three hours in a mixture of one gallon of water and one cup of dishwashing detergent.

Weight for results. Resistive exercise—when force is exerted against a weight—can be applied to the sphincter muscles of the urethra and rectum, which are important to regaining continence, says Wells. Cones that are about the size of a tampon and that come in varying weights are designed for use in the vagina (women) or rectum (men). When a cone is inserted, the sphincter muscles must contract in order to hold the weight and not let it drop.

EXERCISES FOR INCONTINENCE

The pelvic floor is a set of muscles at the bottom of the pelvis that supports the lower internal organs, such as the bladder and uterus, and controls the sphincter muscles, which are the muscles that control the urethra and rectum. When you stop and start your urine stream, you're working these muscles. When this set of muscles becomes weak, incontinence may occur. Since these muscles can be controlled voluntarily, exercises may help strengthen them and in turn help control leakage, especially in cases of stress incontinence. This is true only if the exercises are done properly, however.

Here are a few simple exercises recommended by Help for Incontinent People (HIP) that should be done on a daily basis for best results. If you need additional instruction, HIP can provide manuals and tapes, or you can consult your doctor. In addition, your doctor may recommend exercises of increasing difficulty, depending on your specific case.

1. Lie on your back with your knees bent and feet slightly apart. Contract all the openings in the pelvic floor—the rectum, urethra, and, in women, the vagina, too. To help you isolate the muscles, first squeeze as if trying to keep from passing gas. Then (for women) contract the vagina as if trying not to lose a tampon. Then, proceed forward as if trying to stop urinating. Hold the tension while slowly counting to three. Then slowly release the tension. Repeat five to ten times. You should feel a "lift" inside you. Be sure to breathe smoothly and comfortably and do not tense your stomach, thigh, or buttocks muscles; otherwise, you may be exercising the wrong muscles. Check your abdomen with your hand to make sure the stomach area is relaxed.

2. Repeat the first exercise while using a low stool to support the lower part of your legs. Raising your legs will help further relax the pelvic-floor muscles for the exercise.

3. Third, repeat the first exercise while kneeling on the floor with your elbows resting on a cushion. In this position, the stomach muscles are completely relaxed. If you are unable to kneel, roll up a blanket and place it under your groin while you lie on your stomach.

"Over a few months and with progressive use of the varying weights, the pelvic-floor muscles should get stronger," says Jeter. These weight sets are available from physicians, who can guide your use of the cones, or from medical-supply stores. Be sure to carefully read and follow the accompanying instructions on proper use for best results. Start by holding in the lightest weight for 15 minutes, two times a day. Once successful at that weight, try the next heaviest weight for the same amount of time. Some versions of these cones come with an electronic biofeedback system, called a perineometer, which reports on the amount of pressure you're applying to the inserted cone.

Take control of your muscles every day. To prevent leakage, contract the pelvic-floor muscles when coughing or sneezing. Contract them when carrying or lifting something, too. Do so by standing close to the object to be lifted with your feet slightly apart, one foot just in front of the other. Then, bend your knees but keep your back straight. Lean forward slightly as you contract, or tighten, your pelvic muscles. Then lift the object.

Be wary of exercise gimmicks. Carefully investigate any exercise contraption that claims to help decrease incontinence. A company may promote the fact that its gadget will tone the pelvic-floor muscles, but the device may actually exercise an unrelated muscle group, if it does anything at all. An exerciser for use between the thighs, for instance, will not strengthen the pelvic-floor muscles. If you're not sure if a certain exerciser will benefit your incontinence problem, don't waste your time or money. Check first with your health-care provider.

Make a phone call. Call 1-800-BLADDER, a toll-free number sponsored by HIP, for details on how to receive a free packet of information on services and products for incontinent people.

LACTOSE INTOLERANCE

10 Ways to Manage It

Many folks relish the thought of downing a frosty-cold glass of milk, polishing off a bowl of creamy ice cream, or biting into a piping-hot slice of cheesy pizza. For close to 50 million Americans, though, the aftereffects of indulging in these dairy delights may force them to forgo such foods or suffer some decidedly unpleasant consequences.

The common condition these people share is lactose intolerance. That means they don't properly digest lactose, which is milk sugar found in all milk products. This problem is usually due to a shortage of the enzyme lactase, which normally breaks down milk sugar in the small intestine into simple parts that can be absorbed into the bloodstream. The end result of this lactase deficiency may be gas, stomach pains, bloating, and diarrhea. The severity of the symptoms varies from person to person.

Who is lactose intolerant? It's not an equal opportunity problem. It affects some ethnic groups much more than others. The National Institute of Diabetes & Digestive & Kidney Diseases estimates that 75 percent of African-American, Jewish, Native-American, and Mexican-American adults and 90 percent of Asian-American adults have this condition. Only about 10 to 15 percent of adult Caucasians are lactase deficient, says David Alpers, M.D., a professor of medicine and chief of the Gastroenterology Division at Washington University School of Medicine in St. Louis. Though you may not fall into any of these categories, keep in mind that as we get older, we all lose some of the ability to digest lactose in milk.

Some people figure out that they are lactose intolerant on their own; for others, it takes a trip to a doctor to pinpoint the problem. "Among the black or Asian community, it's kind of folk wisdom that these people don't do well with milk, so they tend not to drink as much," says Alpers. On the other hand, he says, "There's also a significant number of people who are having symptoms from milk sugar and really have no idea of what the problem is."

If you suspect you may be lactose intolerant but you're not sure, it may be worth a visit to a physician to rule out other possible problems (see "Hello, Doctor?" on page 158). Once you know that you are indeed lactose intolerant, you may want to follow these helpful tips to ease your symptoms:

Determine your level of lactose intolerance. The degree of intolerance differs with each person. The easiest way to do this is first to get all lactose out of your system. "That means having no dairy food and no lactose for about three to four weeks," says Jane Zukin, author of *The Dairy-*

HELLO, DOCTOR?

If you're feeling digestive distress that you think may be lactose intolerance but you're not certain, try this simple test. Lay off all milk products for a few weeks and see if your gut gets better. If things don't improve, it may be time to check in with your doctor. Other glitches in the digestive system may be causing your problems. For instance, you may have irritable bowel syndrome, another common digestive disorder that can produce symptoms similar to lactose intolerance. "Another thing that lactose intolerance can be confused with is an intolerance to caffeine," says David Alpers, M.D. So play it safe and get an expert's opinion. It is especially important to consult your doctor if you notice a major change in bowel patterns.

Free Cookbook and editor of *The Newsletter for People with Lactose Intolerance and Milk Allergies.* Then start with very small quantities of milk or cheese. Monitor your symptoms to see how much or how little dairy food you can handle. Once you know your limits, management becomes a little easier.

Stick with small servings. While you may not be able to tolerate an eight-ounce glass of milk all at once, you may feel fine drinking a third of a cup in the morning, a third of a cup in the afternoon, and a third of a cup at night. "If you have 'x' amount of lactase enzyme in your body that can only digest 'x' amount of lactose, it will be easier if you take in less lactose over a longer period of time than if you overload," says Zukin.

Don't eat dairy foods alone. If you eat some cheese or drink some milk, do so with a meal or snack. "Having more in your stomach to digest slows the digestive process and may ease your symptoms," says Zukin.

Color your milk chocolate. A study by researcher Chong Lee at the University of Rhode Island in Kingston found that 35 lactose-intolerant people digested more lactose when they drank milk with cocoa and sugar added than they did when they drank plain milk. They also experienced less bloating and fewer cramps. No one is sure why this is

HIDDEN SOURCES OF LACTOSE

Lactose lurks in many prepared foods. Bread, cereals, pancakes, chocolate, soups, puddings, salad dressings, sherbet, instant cocoa mix, candies, frozen dinners, cookie mixes, and hot dogs may all contain lactose. While the amounts of lactose may be small, people with low tolerance levels can be bothered. "People need to read every single label and be careful of what they eat," says author Jane Zukin. When perusing ingredient labels, it's not just milk that you have to watch for. Whey, curds, milk by-products, dry milk solids, nonfat dry milk powder, casein, galactose, skim milk powder, milk sugar, and whey protein concentrate are all buzzwords that indicate the presence of lactose.

so, but Alpers says it may be because "chocolate delays the emptying of your stomach." A slower emptying rate may mean fewer symptoms.

Supplement your diet. Lactase-enzyme supplements can supply your body with some of what it lacks. They're sold in tablet or liquid form, without a prescription. The tablets are chewed with or right after you consume a dairy product; you add the drops directly to milk. "These work quite well for some people," says Zukin. You can also try lactose-reduced milk.

Try yogurt. "By and large, lactose intolerant people tolerate yogurt pretty well," says Alpers. This holds true, however, only for yogurt with active cultures, which you may have to buy in a health-food store. If you can tolerate yogurt, it's to your advantage to include it in your diet, because this creamy food is a great source of calcium.

Choose hard cheeses. If you find yourself drawn to the cheese aisle, pick hard, aged cheeses such as Swiss, cheddar, or Colby, advises Elyse Sosin, R.D., Supervisor of Clinical Nutrition at Mount Sinai Medical Center in New York. They contain less lactose than soft cheeses.

Avoid processed foods. Lactose is used in a lot of processed foods where you might not expect to find it (see "Hidden Sources of Lactose"). "It's best for people to stick to as much fresh food as possible, and skip the cans, frozen foods, and stuff that comes out of a box," says Zukin. One added benefit to this strategy: You'll be eating a healthier diet.

Get calcium from other foods. Lactose intolerant people, especially women and children, should make sure their calcium intake doesn't plunge. Green, leafy vegetables, such as collard greens, kale, turnip greens, and chinese cabbage (bok choy), as well as oysters, sardines, canned salmon with the bones, and tofu, provide lots of calcium. If your diet is calcium poor, you may want to take calcium supplements; talk to your doctor for a recommendation on proper dosage.

Watch out for medications. Lactose is used as a filler in more than 20 percent of prescription drugs (including many types of birth control pills) and in about 6 percent of over-the-counter medicines. This may not matter to someone who takes medication only occasionally, but Zukin says, "for the person who takes medication on a regular basis, this can be a problem." Complicating matters is the fact that lactose may not be listed under the inactive ingredients on the label. To find out if what you're taking contains lactose, Zukin advises first seeking help from your doctor. You might also check with your pharmacist or write directly to the drug manufacturer.

MENOPAUSE

11 Tips for Coping with "the Change"

For most women, menopause, the cessation of the menstrual cycle, is fraught with rumor and misinformation. Stories of menopausal hot flashes, vaginal dryness, wrinkles, weight gain, depression, anxiety, thinning hair, and loss of sex drive may have you dreading "the change." Relax. Most of the stories you've heard probably aren't true.

Too often, women confuse natural aging changes with menopause. The few symptoms actually associated with the hormonal changes during menopause can usually be handled with a few minor lifestyle changes. Contrary to what most women have heard about menopause, it's a natural period of transition that gives rise to an exciting and challenging period in life.

Menopause is a period of four or five years, usually two years before the last menstrual period and two to three years after it. For most women, menopause occurs between the ages of 45 and 53, although some women experience it earlier and others go through it at a later age. A woman generally experiences menopause at about the same age as her mother did.

Menopause begins with changes in the menstrual cycle—shorter or longer periods, heavier or lighter bleeding, decreased or increased premenstrual symptoms—until the menstrual periods cease altogether. Women should keep track of their irregular bleeding so their physician can help them determine whether these changes are normal or whether they indicate some abnormal changes in the uterine lining.

Although there is much talk about menopausal "symptoms," the only symptoms that have been clearly demonstrated to be associated with the hormonal changes of menopause are hot flashes and vaginal dryness. Mood swings or depression aren't related to hormonal changes as much as they are to fatigue caused from sleep disturbances due to hot flashes, according to Amanda Clark, M.D., assistant professor of obstetrics and gynecology at Oregon Health Sciences University in Portland. "The hormonal fluctuations of menopause aren't believed to cause any major psychological depression," she says.

But menopause signals more than hormonal changes. It is the doorway to a new life. Postmenopausal women are free of the discomforts of menstruation, free of the need for contraceptives, and, in many cases, free of child-rearing responsibilities. For the first time, many women find they can concentrate on their own agendas and do the things they want to do.

Here are some tips about how to make the most of this exciting transition called menopause:

Dress for hot flashes. Eight in ten women experience periods of sudden, intense heat and sweating often called "flushes" or "hot flashes," according to Sadja Greenwood,

ESTROGEN REPLACEMENT THERAPY

Many physicians recommend that women take hormones to make up for the decrease in estrogen levels that occurs during menopause. Estrogen replacement therapy, or ERT (also called hormone replacement therapy or HRT), can reduce or eliminate the hot flashes and vaginal soreness and, in some women, decrease the risk of osteoporosis, says Sadja Greenwood, M.D.

However, ERT isn't without risk. Some studies have shown ERT may increase the risk of developing cancer of the breast and uterus. Amanda Clark, M.D., says studies have shown the increased risk of breast cancer is quite small and that the increased risk of uterine cancer from estrogen replacement can be eliminated by adding the hormone progestin.

Women who have had any of the following are generally not recommended for ERT: cancer of the breast or uterus; ovarian cancer; clots in the legs, pelvis, or lungs; high blood pressure; diabetes; gallstones or gallbladder disease; or large uterine fibroids.

Clark believes that, for most women, the benefits of hormone replacement therapy outweigh the risks. "Fourteen studies have shown that hormone replacement therapy helps prevent heart disease," she says. "Estrogen also helps maintain calcium uptake, which helps prevent osteoporosis."

Greenwood says women should thoroughly discuss the pros and cons of ERT with their physicians. If a woman opts for ERT, Greenwood says, she should take the lowest dose possible and be sure the doctor prescribes a combination of both estrogen and progestin to reduce the risk of uterine cancer.

M.D., an assistant clinical professor in the Department of Obstetrics, Gynecology, and Reproductive Sciences at the University of California at San Francisco. "Hot flashes are the body's response to lower-than-usual estrogen levels," says Greenwood. She recommends wearing loose clothing that is easily removed, such as cardigan sweaters.

Douse it. If you're at home or in a place where it's convenient, you can "spritz" your face with a spray of cool water from a squeeze bottle or you can blot your face with a cool washcloth or moist towelette.

Avoid caffeine and alcohol. If hot flashes seem to be triggered by caffeine and alcohol consumption, Greenwood advises women to avoid them completely. Try substituting noncaffeinated teas or decaffeinated coffee for caffeinated beverages. (Keep in mind that caffeine withdrawal may cause headaches and fatigue for several days.) Greenwood says excess caffeine also causes the kidneys to excrete more calcium, a factor in bone thinning in postmenopausal women.

Carry a personal fan. Many women find they can get relief from the sudden heat of hot flashes by using a small personal fan. Inexpensive wood and paper fans or battery-powered personal fans are small enough to be carried in a purse and can be used anywhere.

Take your time with lovemaking. Hormonal changes associated with menopause often cause a woman's vaginal mucous membranes to become thin and secrete less moisture. The result can be painful sexual intercourse. Some of this lack of moisture can be overcome by taking more time to make love, according to Lonnie Barbach, Ph.D., a nationally recognized sex expert and author of numerous books on the topic. Barbach also suggests exploring other ways of pleasuring one another in addition to intercourse.

Use creams or lubricants. If patient lovemaking doesn't produce enough lubrication for the woman, Clark suggests using lubricating jellies (available in pharmacies), plain vegetable oil, or unscented cold cream. "One of the best lubricants is a product called Astroglide, because it's most like natural secretions," she says. "Jellies like K-Y Jelly are good, but Vaseline tends to be messy and gummy."

Exercise regularly. Menopause has been erroneously linked with depression. Several studies have found that women between the ages of 45 and 55 have no increase in susceptibility to depression. Mood swings during this time may have more to do with a woman's changing role and her self-concept and the physical changes of aging she's experiencing. "For many women," says Clark, "menopause is a milestone, a negative milestone, in their lives. They find the idea of menopause depressing. We need to discard those old ideas." Regular, aerobic exercise such as brisk walking does much to increase the general health level, fight fatigue, and raise the spirits. Exercise also appears to slow changes like loss of strength that many believe to be age related but are actually more associated with a sedentary lifestyle.

Regular, weight-bearing exercises such as walking or jogging can also help stave off the bone thinning of osteoporosis, a problem for many menopausal women. Clark says bones get stronger with regular exercise no matter what your age. "Any weight-bearing exercise is good," says Clark. "But it has to be a weight-bearing exercise, not like swimming, to increase bone density."

Get support. "Another term for menopause is 'climacteric,'" says Susan Woodruff, B.S.N., childbirth and parenting education coordinator at Tuality Community Hospital in Hillsboro, Oregon. "That word applies because it is a really big change. You're closing one chapter in your life and moving on. You may notice body changes—new aches, pains, wrinkles. Menopause is one of life's major change signals. It's helpful to talk to other women about these changes."

Woodruff recommends joining a menopause support group sponsored by a local hospital or community college. Or you might want to form your own group with friends who are experiencing menopause. "Menopause affects how you see yourself, your self-concept, because your roles in life are changing at this time," says Woodruff. "A support group of other women who understand can really help you see yourself as a strong person experiencing a natural life change."

Get plenty of calcium. "Everyone loses calcium as they get older," says Clark. "But in women, as estrogen levels decline, the rate of bone loss increases."

Sonja Connor, M.S., R.D., research associate professor in the School of Medicine at Oregon Health Sciences University in Portland, says, "At menopause, there's an outpouring of calcium in response to the lower estrogen levels. Unless you have really good stores of calcium already, during this time you're going to have an increased need for calcium."

Clark says postmenopausal women taking hormone replacement need 1,000 milligrams of elemental calcium

CALCIUM-RICH FOODS

Calcium is important at any age, but it becomes even more important for menopausal women in order to prevent the bone thinning of osteoporosis. Include these calcium-rich foods in your diet to ensure you're getting enough of this important mineral.

• Almonds • Brewer's yeast • Cheese (opt for nonfat or low-fat varieties) • Dandelion greens • Ice milk or ice cream (opt for lower-fat varieties) • Kelp • Mackerel, canned • Milk (opt for skim or low-fat) • Mustard greens • Oysters • Salmon, canned with bones • Sardines, canned with bones • Soybean curd (tofu) • Yogurt (opt for nonfat or low-fat)

daily; women not taking hormones need 1,500 milligrams of elemental calcium.

Dairy products are good sources of calcium, although you'll be doing yourself an even bigger favor if you choose those that are low in fat, such as skim milk, nonfat yogurt, and low-fat cheeses. For example, an eight-ounce glass of whole milk and an eight-ounce glass of skim milk contain the same amount of elemental calcium (350 milligrams), but the whole milk contains about 70 calories more from fat. To add to your calcium stores, eat a diet that is also rich in vegetables, fruits, and complex carbohydrates (see "Calcium-Rich Foods").

If your diet isn't calcium rich or if your stores of calcium are seriously depleted from a lifetime of poor eating habits, Clark suggests taking calcium supplements. Keep in mind that the number of milligrams of calcium listed on the label of a supplement may not reflect the amount of elemental calcium in the product. For example, it takes 1,200 milligrams of calcium carbonate to get 500 milligrams of elemental calcium. Ask your doctor or pharmacist for advice on choosing a calcium supplement.

Eat a balanced, low-fat diet. Women at menopause not only have an increased risk of osteoporosis, they may also be at risk for heart disease. "At menopause, women's levels of LDL, or so-called 'bad' cholesterol, go up," explains Connor. "Within about ten years, they have the same risk for heart disease as men."

Connor says diet can go a long way toward preventing serious health problems like osteoporosis, cancer, and heart disease in menopausal women. "Diets high in animal products and salt cause the body to excrete more calcium, which contributes to osteoporosis," she says. "Menopausal women should eat less animal protein and less salt. If they switch to more foods from the vegetable kingdom and more complex carbohydrates, they'll be getting less fat [high-fat diets are related to some cancers and heart disease], more calcium, and more of the anti-cancer elements like beta carotene."

Plan for menopause. "The problem," says Connor, "is that most women eat the typical American diet: 40 percent of calories from fat, 20 percent from sugar, and 5 percent from alcohol—essentially empty calories. That means they're getting nutrients from only 35 percent of their calories. On top of that, they don't do any regular exercise. When menopause comes, they need medical intervention in the form of hormone therapy just to catch up with what they've done to their bodies all these years."

Connor believes only a small percentage of women would need hormone therapy if they'd anticipate menopause by eating right and exercising regularly for at least 20 years before the onset of menopause. "Prevention is the best thing," she says. "A lifelong lifestyle of low-fat eating, not smoking, and exercising regularly will usually get you ready to face menopausal changes without any problems." And, of course, no matter what stage in life you're in, it's never too late to benefit from switching to a healthier lifestyle.

MENSTRUAL CRAMPS
6 Ways to Tackle Them

Three weeks out of each month you feel great. But then comes your period, and with it, those awful cramps. You try to ignore them and go about your daily business, but the pain and discomfort continue to divert your attention. For most women, menstrual cramps last no more than one or two days each month. But this can seem endless when you're trying to function normally. And the congestive, bloating-type symptoms that often accompany these cramps may only compound the problem.

"Primary menstrual cramps are hereditary," says Phyllis Frey, A.R.N.P., a nurse practitioner at Bellegrove OB-GYN, Inc., in Bellevue, Washington. "There is no specific cause determined. It just seems that during your period, your uterus cramps up and your sensitivity to that cramping is pretty acute," she explains.

"Sometimes, primary cramps will lessen after giving birth," says Harold Zimmer, M.D., an obstetrician and gynecologist in Bellevue, Washington. "We are not sure why this is, but it could be that the stretching out of the cervix during delivery reduces the pulling against it that can occur when the uterus contracts or cramps up," he adds.

"Secondary menstrual cramps, on the other hand, are caused by some underlying condition, such as pelvic infection, pelvic lesions, fibroids, endometriosis, bad pelvic congestion, or pelvic varicose veins," says Zimmer. "They are usually a little worse than primary cramps, depending on how significant the underlying condition is," he adds.

In either case, menstrual cramps are usually the result of a prostaglandin excess. Prostaglandin is a hormone produced by the uterine lining that mediates many processes within the body. It can bring on headaches, intestinal cramps, and labor, according to Zimmer. While secondary cramps are usually treated by curing the underlying condition, primary cramps are largely self-treatable with over-the-counter medications and some basic comfort measures. Here are some suggestions:

Take ibuprofen or aspirin. "These medications help to lower the level of prostaglandins, which can lessen or alleviate the cramps," says Zimmer. "These drugs also cost much less than those that a doctor would prescribe for cramps," adds Frey.

Hold a heating pad to the cramped area. "The heat will relax the muscles and soften the pain of the cramping," says Frey. "It works best if you can lie down at the same time," she says.

HELLO, DOCTOR?

All of these experts agree that if you notice your cramps getting more severe, or if you've never had menstrual cramps before and suddenly develop them, it is time to visit your doctor. "Women with primary menstrual cramps start having them when they first begin menstruating or within one to two years of the onset of menstruation," says Harold Zimmer, M.D. "So if you notice a significant change, you should be evaluated to see if there is some secondary cause for the cramps," he continues.

"Secondary cramps also tend to be pretty mean cramps that are often accompanied by nausea, vomiting, and even diarrhea," says Phyllis Frey, A.R.N.P. "They can also occur with backache and pain down the thighs."

The causes for secondary cramps could include endometriosis (the presence of endometrial tissue in places where it is not usually found), pelvic congestion, pelvic varicose veins, pelvic infection, or fibroids (benign tumors in the uterine wall). "Secondary cramps caused by fibroids tend to occur during actual ovulation, while those caused by endometriosis may be present throughout the month," says Zimmer. "With pelvic congestion or pelvic veins, the cramps tend to occur four or five days before the menstrual flow itself," he adds. While you may get some relief from secondary cramps with self-treatment, the underlying conditions that cause them really need to be treated by a physician. And Zimmer warns that exercising may actually worsen secondary cramps.

Maintain a regular aerobic exercise program. "This doesn't mean you have to exercise through an episode of cramps. Keeping up a regular exercise or fitness program the rest of the month seems to make these episodes less intense when they do occur," says Frey. "Exercising also increases pelvic circulation, which helps to clear out the excess prostaglandins a little faster," adds Zimmer.

Take a hot bath. "Just as with a heating pad, a hot bath relaxes the muscles and increases circulation to the pelvic area," says Zimmer. It can also relieve some of the lower back pain that can accompany cramps.

Do some pelvic-tilt exercises. "Getting down on all fours, bringing the elbows to the ground, and rocking back and forth tends to help some women," says Zimmer. "It works especially well for women with a retroverted uterus [one that is more swollen and puts more pressure on the back]," he adds.

Talk to your doctor about birth control pills. "Birth control pills help to suppress ovulation, which lessens the severity of menstrual cramps," says Zimmer. "It is really not certain why they help so much," adds Frey. "It could be that by lessening the flow and length of a woman's period, the cramps are lessened as well," she continues. Birth control pills are not without side effects, however, and certain women should not use them, so be sure to discuss them thoroughly with your doctor.

MORNING SICKNESS

13 Ways to Ease the Queasiness

The nausea and vomiting of early pregnancy were written about as early as 2000 B.C. Unfortunately, the ancient Egyptians didn't have a cure for the condition, either.

Some 50 to 70 percent of American women will suffer from nausea or vomiting, or both, during the first three months (also known as the first trimester) of their pregnancies. The severity and even occurrence vary not only from woman to woman, but from pregnancy to pregnancy in the same individual.

Some women never have even the slightest touch of queasiness. Some are ill in the morning and recover by lunch. And some stay sick all day for days on end, wondering why it's called "morning sickness" when it lasts 24 hours.

No one knows what causes morning sickness. It is less common among Eskimos and native African tribes than in Western civilizations. But today's doctors emphasize it's not psychological, as was once believed. "Morning sickness is not a psychological rejection of the pregnancy," says Donald R. Coustan, M.D., professor and chair of obstetrics-gynecology at Brown University School of Medicine and chief of obstetrics-gynecology at Women and Infants Hospital of Rhode

HELLO, DOCTOR?

If morning sickness persists past the third month or you find yourself so ill that you're losing weight, see your physician. Watch out, too, for becoming dehydrated; you'll feel dizzy when you stand, or your urine output will be scanty and dark colored.

Island in Providence. "It is not a symbolic attempt to vomit up the baby."

Since hormones run amok during early pregnancy, researchers theorize that these abnormal hormone levels contribute somehow to the existence of morning sickness. A suspected culprit is human chorionic gonadotropin (HCG), the hormone tested in home pregnancy kits, which hits an all-time high in those first months. But other hormones may play a role as well. High levels of progesterone, for example, result in smooth-muscle relaxation, slowing down the digestive process, says Cheryl Coleman, R.N., B.S.N., I.C.C.E., a childbirth educator at Hillcrest Medical Center in Tulsa, Oklahoma, and director of public relations for the International Childbirth Education Association.

"There are a lot of changes going on in the pregnant woman's body," points out Kermit E. Krantz, M.D., university distinguished professor, professor of gynecology and obstetrics, and professor of anatomy at the University of Kansas Medical Center in Kansas City. "Your kidneys increase their activity by 100 percent. Your blood volume will increase by 50 percent."

If you're suffering from morning sickness, you probably don't care what causes it. You just want relief. Time will eventually take care of it; the condition usually subsides after the third month. (Scant words of comfort.) While you're waiting, however, here's what the experts suggest you try for relief:

Don't worry about crumbs in the sheets. Keep crackers by the bed. Eating a few low-sodium crackers as soon as you wake up—and before you get out of bed—is the first line of defense against morning sickness.

Graze. Eat frequent, small meals. You may want to eat five to six times a day. Sometimes, hunger pangs bring on

THE BRIGHT SIDE

The good news about morning sickness? (You doubt that there's anything good to say about this subject?) Studies have shown that women who experience nausea and vomiting early in their pregnancies are more likely to deliver full-term, healthy babies.

Researchers in Colorado Springs, Colorado, and Albany, New York, studied 414 pregnant women. Nearly 90 percent said they had some of the symptoms of morning sickness. But these women were more likely to carry their pregnancies to full term and deliver a live baby than the women who had no morning sickness at all. On the other hand, don't panic if you don't experience morning sickness. Plenty of women sail through pregnancy without nausea and deliver healthy babies.

the feelings of nausea. That's because acids in the stomach have nothing to digest when there's no food around.

Don't drink and eat at the same time. In other words, drink your fluids between meals, instead of during meals, to avoid too much bulk in the stomach, says Krantz.

Fill up on fluids. You need at least eight glasses a day, says Krantz. "Avoiding dehydration is most important, especially in the summertime."

Go for a liquid diet. You may find it easier on your tummy to emphasize liquids over solids, says Coustan. Get your nutrients from bouillon, juices, and other liquids.

Stick to bland foods. This isn't the time to try that new Thai restaurant. Spicy foods just don't cut it right now.

Choose complex carbohydrates. Pasta, bread, potatoes—the foods you think of as starches—are easier to digest and they're soothing, says Coleman.

Avoid fatty foods. Fats are harder to digest than carbohydrates or proteins, explains Coleman.

Don't sniff. Certain odors often trigger the feelings of nausea. "Pay attention to what these triggers are and avoid them," suggests Coustan. "Let someone else do the cooking if that bothers you, for example."

Avoid sudden moves. Don't change your posture quickly. "Don't sit up in bed too suddenly," advises Krantz. "Get up easily."

Take vitamin B₆. A number of physicians recommend this vitamin for morning sickness because of its ability to fight nausea. Talk to your doctor before trying a supplement, however, and be sure not to exceed 25 milligrams of the vitamin each day.

Take a hike. OK, go for a walk outside every day. "It's a positive thing you can do for yourself," says Coleman. "And the exercise and fresh air may make you feel better." Be sure to check with your doctor before trying anything more strenuous than a stroll, however.

Don't forget to brush. If you do succumb to vomiting, take good care of your teeth and brush afterwards. Otherwise, the frequent contact with the harsh acids in what you throw up can eat away at tooth enamel.

NAUSEA AND VOMITING

9 Soothing Strategies

Perhaps it's the 24-hour flu bug, or maybe it was something you ate. Whatever the cause, now you're feeling queasy and sick.

The tips that follow are designed to reduce your discomfort and to help your symptoms go away as quickly as possible. If vomiting is violent or persists for more than 24 hours or if your vomit contains blood, see a physician without delay.

Evaluate the cause and treat the symptoms accordingly. Nausea and vomiting are two vague symptoms that can be caused by many illnesses, says Albert B. Knapp, M.D., an adjunct assistant attending physician at Lenox Hill Hospital in New York. If you suspect your symptoms are due to a headache or to morning sickness, for example, be sure to also read the section in this book that corresponds to that particular illness.

Stick to clear liquids. Your stomach probably doesn't need the added burden of digesting food, says Knapp. He recommends sticking to fluids until you feel a little better. "If you are vomiting, do not start fluids until the vomiting has stopped," he says. "Then start with warm fluids, since cold ones can irritate the stomach. The fluid should have sugar in it. The sugar helps absorption." Liquids are easier to digest and are necessary to prevent the dehydration that may occur from vomiting, according to Cornelius P. Dooley, M.D., a gastroenterologist in Santa Fe, New Mexico. He recommends diluted, noncitrus fruit juices.

Let it run its course. The best cure for the 24-hour stomach flu is bed rest mixed with a tincture of time, doctors agree. "You'll feel miserable, but you've got to let it run its course," says Dooley.

Don't drink alcohol. Alcohol can be very irritating to the stomach. The same goes for fatty foods, highly seasoned foods, caffeine, and cigarettes.

Stick to easy-to-digest foods. When you are ready to start eating again, start with soft foods, such as bread, unbuttered toast, steamed fish, or bananas, says Neville R. Pimstone, M.D., chief of hepatology in the Division of Gastroenterology at the University of California at Davis. "Avoid fats, and stick to a low-fiber diet," he says. What about chicken soup? "Chicken soup probably has too much fat," Pimstone says. Start with very small amounts of food and slowly build up to larger meals, says Steven C. Fiske, M.D., assistant clinical professor of medicine and gastroenterology at the University of Medicine and Dentistry of New Jersey in Newark.

Let it flow. The worst thing you can do for vomiting is to fight it, says Knapp. Trying to hold back the urge can actually cause tears in your esophagus.

Take Pepto-Bismol. Over-the-counter stomach medications that contain bismuth, such as Pepto-Bismol, may coat the stomach and relieve discomfort, says Pimstone. However, he advises against taking Alka-Seltzer, which contains aspirin and may irritate the stomach.

Try a cold compress. A cold compress on your head can be very comforting when you are vomiting, says Knapp.

Maintain your electrolyte balance. Along with replacing fluids, it is also important to maintain the balance of sodium and potassium (known as electrolytes) in your system, says Fiske. He recommends a sports drink, such as Gatorade, which is easy on the stomach and is designed to replace both fluids and electrolytes.

OILY HAIR

5 Tips for Cutting the Grease

You wash and style your hair every morning, but within a few short hours, it looks stringy and dirty. You, like millions of others, have oily hair.

A certain amount of oil secretion from oil glands on the scalp is healthy and necessary. Sebum, the natural oil produced by the oil glands, protects your hair shafts from breaking. Oil also gives your hair luster and shine. But, let's face it, with oily hair, you've got too much of a good thing.

Oily hair is a second cousin to oily skin, according to Nelson Lee Novick, M.D., associate clinical professor of dermatology at the Mount Sinai School of Medicine in New York. "The oil is just coming up on a different part of the skin," he says. "It's usually a genetic problem. But at certain times, most people have oilier hair due to fluctuations in hormones."

Women often complain of oilier hair at the beginning and end of the menstrual cycle. Paul Contorer, M.D., chief of dermatology for Kaiser Permanente and clinical professor of dermatology at Oregon Health Sciences University in Portland, says that for many people, oily hair begins at puberty: "We often see teenagers with oily hair because the androgen hormones stimulate the sebaceous glands to produce more oil."

While you can't change your genes or your hormones, you can do some things to control your oily locks.

Shampoo often. "People with oily hair can shampoo every day," says Contorer. "Keep in mind that hair is just dead protein. Washing often won't hurt it."

Use a "no-nonsense" shampoo. Often, shampoos have all kinds of additives and conditioners in them. People with oily hair need a good solvent-type shampoo, one that will cut the grease, says Contorer. "I tell my patients to add a couple of drops of Ivory Liquid to their shampoo," he says. If you don't like the idea of putting dishwashing liquid on your head, there are plenty of commercial shampoos that will cut through the excess oil, says Rose Dygart, owner of Le Rose Salon of Beauty in Lake Oswego, Oregon, and a cosmetologist and barber who has been teaching and practicing hair care for 35 years. "Look for a castile-type soap without conditioning additives," she advises. "Commercial products like Prell and Suave do a good job on oily hair." Dygart says normal hair needs a shampoo with a pH between 4.5 and 6.7, but oily hair requires a more alkaline product. Look for shampoos with a pH higher than 6.7, she says.

Rinse thoroughly. Whatever shampoo you use, be sure you rinse thoroughly. Soap residue will only collect dirt and oil more quickly, says Novick.

Forget conditioners. Conditioners coat the hair, which is something that oily hair doesn't need, says Dygart. Apply a small amount of conditioner only to the ends if they've become dried out.

Try an acidic rinse. One way to decrease the oil is to rinse with diluted vinegar or lemon juice after shampooing. Dygart says to use two tablespoons of white vinegar to one cup of water or use the juice of one lemon (strained) to one cup of water. Rinse the mixture through your hair, then rinse your hair with warm water.

OILY SKIN

10 Ways to Cope

You may welcome the shine from the sun, but, if you have oily skin, you probably dread the shine on your cheeks and forehead. Just as some people are born with dry skin, others are born with overly oily skin. "Oily skin is basically a genetic problem," says Margaret Robertson, M.D., a dermatologist in private practice in Lake Oswego, Oregon. "If your mother or father had oily skin, chances are good that you will, too."

Hormones also play a big part. "We often see people with oily skin who are in their teens or early 20s, people who are undergoing hormonal changes," says Nelson Lee Novick, M.D., associate clinical professor of dermatology at Mount Sinai School of Medicine in New York.

But oily skin doesn't just affect teenagers and young adults. Many women notice oily skin problems during pregnancy, around the time of their menstrual periods, or at menopause. Even some types of birth control pills can increase skin oiliness.

One of the biggest myths about oily skin is that it causes acne. "Acne is caused when oil becomes trapped below the skin's pores and becomes contaminated with bacteria," explains Novick. "When you have oily skin, the oil isn't blocked because it's coming to the skin's surface."

The good news about oily skin is that it keeps the skin younger-looking. Over time, people with oily skin tend to wrinkle less than people with dry or normal skin.

While you can't alter your genes or completely control your hormones, there are plenty of things you can do to cope with your oily skin.

Keep your skin squeaky clean. As anyone with oily skin knows, the oilier the skin, the dirtier the skin looks and feels. To help combat this feeling, it's important to keep the skin clean. Vera Brown, skin expert to many of Hollywood's stars and author of *Vera Brown's Natural Beauty Book*, says oily-skinned people should wash the skin at least twice a day.

Dermatologist Paul Contorer, M.D., chief of dermatology at Kaiser Permanente and clinical professor of dermatology at Oregon Health Sciences University in Portland, recommends a detergent-type soap. "I tell my patients with oily skin to mix a couple of drops of dishwashing detergent like Ivory Liquid in with their regular soap," he says. "It's a great solvent for the oil."

HELLO, DOCTOR?

In most cases, oily skin can be treated at home. However, you'll want to call a doctor if:
- You develop acne.
- You notice any sudden change in your skin (if it suddenly goes from dry to oily, for example).

Brown thinks detergent soaps are too harsh even for oily skin and recommends twice-daily cleansing with a glycerine soap instead. If you find detergent soap too irritating for your skin, try the glycerine variety.

Try aloe vera. Brown likes to follow a thorough facial cleansing with pure aloe vera gel (available in health-food stores). "The aloe vera helps absorb oil," she says, "and it helps cleanse the pores." She recommends dabbing the face two to three times a day with cool aloe vera gel (keep it in the refrigerator) and letting it dry.

Wipe with astringents. Contorer says that wiping the oily parts of the face with rubbing alcohol or a combination of alcohol and acetone (such as is found in Seba-Nil Liquid Cleanser) can help dry oiliness. "It's as good and less expensive than those astringents with perfumes in them," he says.

Frank Parker, M.D., professor and chairman of the Department of Dermatology at Oregon Health Sciences University in Portland, says oily-skinned people should wipe the face between washings with alcohol wipes. You can buy premoistened alcohol wipes in the cosmetic department of most stores. Novick recommends using alcohol, too, but he prefers the convenience of individually wrapped towelettes. "You can carry these with you and wipe the oil off every few hours," he says. "The alcohol acts as a degreaser."

Carry tissues. Novick says if you don't have towelettes, even paper facial tissues can help wipe away excess oils. You can also purchase special oil-absorbing tissues from cosmetics companies that are very effective in removing excess oil between cleansings, says Robertson.

Chill out with cold water rinses. Robertson advises splashing the face a couple of times a day with cold water. "The water is good for getting rid of excess oils, and I prefer it to adding more chemicals to the skin," she says.

Ban moisturizers. While people with dry skin are forever smearing on moisturizers, oily-skinned people shouldn't use them, says Robertson.

Brown agrees. "In all my years of dealing with skin care, I've never seen a moisturizer that's good for oily skin," she says. "Oily-skinned people should never go to bed with cream on their faces."

Novick suggests avoiding the application of oils, too. "Never put mineral oil or petroleum jelly on oily skin," he says. "Applying external oils to oily skin can clog the pores and cause acne."

Mist it. With all the cleansing and wiping, you might be concerned about overdrying the skin. But if you shouldn't use moisturizers, what should you do? Brown says to use a facial mist. "You can buy facial mists in health-food stores," she says. "They're mineral water with herbs and vitamins added. You just spray them onto the face. They add moisture without adding oil or chemicals."

Make a scrub. Brown says scrubs are excellent for removing excess surface oil. She recommends this almond-honey scrub: Mix a small amount of almond meal (ground almonds) with honey. Then gently massage the paste onto your skin with a hot washcloth. Rinse thoroughly. You can also make a scrub from oatmeal mixed with aloe vera, says Brown. Rub gently onto the skin, leave on for 15 minutes, then wash off thoroughly. If you suffer from acne on your face, however, you should probably skip the scrub, since it can aggravate already-irritated skin.

Masque it. Masques applied to the face can reduce oiliness. Brown says you can purchase clay masques or mix Fuller's Earth (available at pharmacies) with a little water to make a paste. Apply to the face and leave on for about 20 minutes before rinsing off.

Use water-based cosmetics. Brown says oily-skinned people should stay away from cosmetics as much as possible. "Try and go without makeup as much as you can," she advises. When you do use makeup, Novick recommends water-based rather than oil-based types. "Go with the powder or gel blushers," he says. "And stay away from cream foundations that add oil."

OSTEOPOROSIS

22 Ways to Combat Brittle Bones

Sometimes it may seem like a losing battle. We're responsible for giving the body all the calcium it needs. When we don't, it takes the bone-building mineral right from the reserves in the bones, "which leads to the breakdown of the bone structure," says Robert P. Heaney, M.D., John A. Creighton University Professor at Creighton University in Omaha, Nebraska.

Osteoporosis, or porous bones, affects many more women than men. There are a number of reasons why this is so. After puberty, males have more bone at most sites than females do, explains Conrad Johnston, M.D., chief of the Division of Endocrinology and Metabolism at Indiana University School of Medicine in Indianapolis. So at peak bone mass, men are at an advantage. What's more, while both men and women begin to lose bone mass as they age, this loss becomes accelerated in women at menopause, when estrogen levels drop. Bone loss in women eventually levels off to about one percent per year, says Johnston. Men begin to lose bone mass sometime around age 45 or 50, he says, but they lose only about half a percent per year. Why men lose bone mass is unclear.

The best prevention: building strong bones now to prevent fractures and other complications later. Here's how to win the war against brittle bones.

Make like Arnold Schwarzenegger. Well, not exactly. But weight lifting is a good way not only to build muscle but bone. "It stimulates the activation of new bone cells," says Richard C. Bozian, M.D., professor of medicine, assistant professor of biochemistry, and director of the Division of Nutrition at the University of Cincinnati. However, before beginning any weight-lifting program, consult your doctor. In general, always start with lighter weights and gradually progress to heavier ones.

Use resistance to make your bones more resistant. "The skeleton is sensitive to mechanical load," says Johnston. Mechanical load is the amount of force you use against your skeleton, and certain activities that use the body's own weight as a force against gravity are the best way to "load up." The result: increased bone-cell production. You can actually see the results of loading in the significantly developed swinging arm of avid tennis and baseball players. "Exercise is one of the most positive things a woman can do to fight osteoporosis," asserts Bozian. While running is a top bone builder, some people find that it packs too much of a punch for their joints. Walking, besides being less stressful to the body, can be done by almost anyone, almost anywhere, without expensive equipment. And "the motion of walking helps the entire body," says Victor G. Ettinger, M.D., medical director of Bone Diagnostic Centres in Torrance and Long Beach, California. As for lower-impact activities, such as swimming and bicycling: "These are helpful, too," says Bozian. No matter which exercise you choose, Johnston recommends that it be performed one hour a day, three days a week for best results. Irony lies in the fact that those who exercise exhaustively, like professional athletes, can suffer from malnutrition. This can lead to a decrease in calcium intake. In women, it can also lead to amenorrhea, or no menstrual cycle, putting them at increased risk for osteoporosis.

Maintain a healthy weight. If you are underweight (say, more than ten percent lighter than the average weight for your age and height), you are at higher risk for a deficiency of calcium and other important vitamins and minerals, which can affect your bones' health. If you are overweight, you may have stronger bones than someone thinner; however, you also may be less active and less likely to follow an exercise routine, which is also important to keeping bones healthy.

Start drinking milk again. Mom was right when she made you drink milk at every meal. In addition to its calcium

HOW TO GET CALCIUM WITHOUT DRINKING MILK

For a variety of reasons, some people don't consume enough dairy products every day to get enough calcium. Dieters, for example, often shun dairy's high fat. Some individuals simply don't like the taste of milk and milk products. And yet others are lactose intolerant, which means their bodies have a hard time digesting dairy foods (see LACTOSE INTOLERANCE). Are these "dairy deserters" destined to a life of brittle bones? Not necessarily. There are many other sources of dietary calcium. To get the most calcium, eat foods in the raw; as foods are cooked, calcium can leach into the cooking water. Here are some nondairy, calcium-rich options:

Orange juice: The calcium fortified variety of orange juice, that is. "This is a wonderful alternative for people who simply don't like milk, because it is fortified to the same extent," says Robert P. Heaney, M.D.

Beans: Kidney and pinto head the list, and for the adventurous, tofu (soybean curd) is calcium- and protein-rich.

Broccoli: Yet another good reason to munch a few stalks—preferably in the raw.

Nuts: Hazelnuts, Brazil nuts, and almonds are among the best choices.

Fruit: Figs and prunes are very high in calcium.

Leafy greens: Romaine lettuce, collards, and kale are good choices. The exception: spinach. "The calcium in spinach is not readily available to the body," explains Heaney.

Salmon and sardines: Both are good sources of calcium. Salmon is also a good source of vitamin D.

And for the lactose intolerant: More and more dairy products made with easily digestible lactic acid are on the market. Lactic acid tablets are also available. And, you shouldn't have a problem with these two dairy products:

Yogurt: The lactose, or sugar, in yogurt, has already been broken down, so your digestive system won't have to do it. Substitute yogurt for sour cream in recipes.

Hard cheeses: The lactose breaks down during the aging process.

content, milk is fortified with vitamin D, and "vitamin D facilitates the absorption of calcium," says Bozian.

THE FACTS ON FLUORIDE

"Fluoride is the only substance we know that actually builds up bones," says Victor G. Ettinger, M.D. "But the problem is, we just don't know how much to give." While fluoride is a bone builder, it is generally believed that too much of it can actually make bones brittle. But even scientific studies have not yielded that same conclusion every time. "Some studies have found that fluoride had no effect on bone-fracture rate," says Conrad Johnston, M.D. "Others have shown a decrease in the amount of fractures suffered by patients." Inconclusive studies are one reason why "the use of fluoride therapeutically, especially in large doses, remains very controversial," Johnston adds.

Through similar tests, drugs containing fluoride have been studied but not approved by the U.S. Food and Drug Administration (FDA). Others, like Didronel, are considered only experimental. Didronel was initially developed as a drug to help those with Paget's disease, a condition in which the bones thicken and soften. The drug was found to build bone, so it is used on a very limited basis to treat osteoporosis. A study, carried out by several medical centers and coordinated through Emory University in Atlanta, has shown a reduction in the rate of fractures in patients who have taken Didronel. However, the drug has been administered over a relatively short period of time and in relatively few patients. As typified by this study, the testing of fluoride drugs continues, so final recommendations about the use of fluoride in treating osteoporosis cannot yet be made by the medical community.

Get some sun. Rays of sunshine activate the vitamin D in the body. Studies have shown that women in Northern Europe and England, for instance, where the weather can be cold and dreary more often than not, have a higher rate of osteoporosis than women who are from warmer, sunnier climates. That doesn't mean you should go out and bake yourself in the sun, however. Fifteen minutes of sun exposure on the hands, arms, and face each day may be all that you need and should not be enough to greatly increase your risk of skin cancer. (Sunscreen, by the way, blocks out the light rays that are responsible for activating vitamin D.) On the other hand, if you are at increased risk of getting skin cancer (because you are fair skinned, for example), your best bet may be to keep your skin protected from sunlight (by avoiding sun exposure altogether or by applying a sunscreen with a sun protection factor [SPF] of 15 or higher) and emphasize dietary sources of vitamin D, such as fortified milk, instead.

Cut down on caffeine. "Caffeine stimulates the loss of calcium through the urine," says Bozian. One study found that drinking more than two cups of average brewed coffee or four cups of average brewed tea per day can increase calcium loss.

Pass up the salt shaker. Salt can also increase the amount of calcium lost through the urine. "The more sodium you excrete, the more calcium you excrete," says Rose Hust, osteoporosis coordinator at the Knoxville Orthopedic Clinic in Tennessee. High-sodium diets may also contribute to osteoporosis in a less direct way, she adds. If you take a diuretic to pull excess salt out of the body, it will also pull out calcium.

Don't worry about phosphorus. There has been some concern that consuming high levels of phosphorus can influence bone loss and risk of osteoporosis. The Food and Drug Administration addressed the issue, however, and found no evidence to substantiate this worry.

Be wise about protein. For healthy bones, protein is a double-edged sword. "Too much protein in the diet can increase calcium excretion," says Hust. However, protein is needed to help maintain a component of bone called collagen, which is made up of proteins. It's not so much a question of eating too much protein, but of not getting enough calcium to balance out the amount of protein in the diet. If you have an adequate calcium intake, you probably don't need to worry about getting too much protein. However, if you don't get much calcium in your diet, you'd be wise to avoid consuming an excess amount of protein.

Schedule your fiber intake. "Fiber can decrease calcium absorption by combining with calcium in the intestine, and at the same time, by increasing the rate at which food is passed through the intestinal tract," explains Hust. But don't eliminate fiber from your diet altogether.

FOR DAIRY LOVERS:
HOW TO USE EVEN MORE

• Use milk instead of water to mix up hot cereals, hot chocolate, and soups.

• Substitute plain yogurt for half the mayonnaise in dressings.

• Top casseroles, omelets, toast, and baked potatoes with low-fat grated or shredded cheese.

• Try low-fat and nonfat varieties of milk, cheese, sour cream, ice cream, and cottage cheese.

• Add skim milk to coffee instead of adding fattening cream or nondairy creamer.

Just try to have calcium-rich foods or calcium supplements between—not during—fiber-rich meals.

Make your own soup. When preparing stock from bones, add a small amount of vinegar to leach the calcium out of the bones. "The amount of calcium in a single pint of homemade soup is equal to the calcium found in a quart or more of milk," says Hust.

Say no to alcohol. Alcohol also interferes with the body's ability to absorb calcium.

Put out that cigarette. "Smoking has been shown to be associated with lower bone mass," says Johnston, since nicotine interferes with calcium absorption.

Check your medicines. Antacids that contain aluminum can interfere with calcium absorption. And some prescription drugs can increase the amount of calcium lost in the urine. For instance, diuretics, which are used to treat hypertension; tetracycline, an antibiotic often used to treat severe cases of acne; and high doses of cortisone drugs or steroids, such as those used to treat arthritis, are a few of the offenders.

Replace your estrogen in menopause. The hormone estrogen is vital to the maintenance of bone. When estrogen levels decrease after menopause, bone loss is "dramatically accelerated," says Ettinger. Estrogen replacement therapy can help slow that calcium drain. Estrogen replacement therapy is not for every woman, however, so be sure to discuss it thoroughly with your doctor.

Carefully consider calcium supplements. "Chances are, if you are a candidate for supplements, your diet is not only low in calcium but in other nutrients the body needs," says Heaney. "Your best bet is to primarily get calcium from the foods you eat." If your doctor recommends that you take a supplement, never exceed 2,500 milligrams per day; excessive calcium can lead to kidney stones. The supplement should be taken between meals with juice instead of water, says Hust. The reason: The vitamin C in fruit juices helps the body absorb calcium.

Get the right amount of calcium. Women, especially, need different amounts of calcium at different times of their lives. The Recommended Daily Allowance (RDA) for females age 11 to 25—the big bone-building years—is 1,200 milligrams. After age 25, the RDA is 800 milligrams; however, the National Institutes of Health recommends 1,000 milligrams after age 25. The RDA for postmenopausal women is 1,500 milligrams, and for pregnant women, it's 2,000 milligrams daily. Men should increase their calcium intake as they age, from 800 milligrams to 1,000 milligrams a day. For both men and women, consuming close to 3,000 milligrams a day can be toxic, says Bozian, and can interfere with the absorption of the vital minerals copper and zinc.

PREMENSTRUAL SYNDROME

11 Ways to Ease the Discomforts

You've heard the joke before. A woman flies off the handle at work or at home and everyone around her chimes in with, "It must be that time of the month again."

The joke, of course, misses the point that women, at times, actually do get upset by their demanding husbands, whiny kids, and stressful jobs. For some women, however, the joke holds more truth than they'd like to believe. For these women, "that time of the month" really is a period of emotional imbalance, anger, depression, and anxiety. Situations that they normally cope well with suddenly become insurmountable. And the energy and health they enjoy most of the time give way to fatigue, achiness, and weight gain almost overnight.

These women have what is known as premenstrual syndrome, or PMS, a condition that has no known cause and no complete cure. But research into the topic has brought about several theories as to what may make some women more vulnerable to PMS.

"The two most widely held theories, neither of which has huge support, include an ovarian hormone imbalance of either estrogen or progesterone and a brain hormone change or deficiency," says Harold Zimmer, M.D., an obstetrician and gynecologist in private practice in Bellevue, Washington. Zimmer stresses that no single cause of PMS has ever been proven and that much of the research is contradictory.

Whatever the cause, the symptoms can include anxiety, irritability, mood swings, and anger; indeed, these symptoms occur in more than 80 percent of women who suffer from PMS. Other symptoms may include sugar cravings, fatigue, headaches, dizziness, shakiness, abdominal bloating, breast tenderness, and overall swelling. Much less common are depression, memory loss, and feelings of isolation. The symptoms, and their severity, vary from woman to woman.

"Symptoms are definitely cyclic, and that is one of the main criteria for diagnosing this condition. And the symptoms generally disappear with the onset of the woman's period," says Phyllis Frey, A.R.N.P., a nurse practitioner at Bellegrove OB-GYN, Inc., in Bellevue, Washington. "It's often the emotional symptoms that bring people in to the doctor," she adds.

As for what you can do to relieve the discomfort of PMS, there are several home remedies. And according to Zimmer, the home remedies probably work as well as, or better than, the medical remedies available. Here's what you can try:

Maintain a well-balanced diet. Include lots of fresh fruits and vegetables, starches, raw seeds and nuts, fish, poultry, and whole grains. "It is just sort of common sense dietary measures," says Zimmer.

Go easy on sugar. Your cravings for sugar may be strong during this time, but giving in to the sugar craving may make you feel even worse and can intensify your feelings of irritability and anxiety. To make fending off your sugar cravings a little easier, try keeping healthy snacks readily available and keeping sugary foods out of reach. If you can't give up the sweets completely, try eating only small amounts at a time, and opt for things like fruits or apple juice that can help satisfy your sugar craving and provide nutrients.

Eat small, frequent meals. You don't want to go long periods without food because that can potentially intensify your premenstrual symptoms as well, says Zimmer.

Avoid alcohol. Both Zimmer and Frey stress that alcohol will only make you feel more depressed and fatigued. Alcohol also depletes the body's stores of B vitamins and minerals and disrupts carbohydrate metabolism. It also disrupts the liver's ability to metabolize hormones, which can lead to higher-than-normal estrogen levels. So if you need to be holding a beverage at that party, try a non-alcoholic cocktail, such as mineral water with a twist of lime or lemon or a dash of bitters.

Cut down on caffeinated beverages. These include coffee, tea, and colas. Caffeine can intensify anxiety, irritability, and mood swings. It may also increase breast tenderness. Try substituting water-processed decaffeinated coffee; grain-based coffee substitutes such as Pero, Postum, and Caffix; and ginger tea.

Cut the fat. Eating too much dietary fat can interfere with liver efficiency. And some beef contains small amounts of synthetic estrogens. Too much protein can also increase the body's demand for minerals. Opt for smaller servings of lean meats, fish or seafood, beans, peas, seeds, and nuts. Use more whole grains, rice, vegetables, and fruits to fill out your meals.

Put down the salt shaker. Table salt and high-sodium foods such as bouillon, commercial salad dressings, catsup, and hot dogs can worsen fluid retention, bloating, and breast tenderness.

Practice stress management. "Learning to control and reduce your level of stress has a great effect on reducing the symptoms of PMS," says Zimmer. Try joining a stress-management or stress-reduction program at your local hospital or community college; learning biofeedback techniques; meditating; exercising; or doing anything that helps you to relax and cope with stress.

Try not to plan big events during your PMS time. "I don't like to encourage my patients to plan their lives around their menstrual cycle, but if they have the option of planning a big social event at some time other than their PMS time, it would help them out to do so," says Zimmer. "The increased stress of the event will only make the PMS symptoms worse," he adds.

Exercise aerobically. "Besides being a great stress reducer, aerobic exercise triggers the release of endorphins (the natural brain opiates) and produces a 'runner's high,'" says Zimmer. "Good forms of aerobic exercise include running, stair-stepping, bicycling, or taking an aerobics class," he continues. "The social environment of a health club can also make you feel better by encouraging you to interact with other people," he adds. He also goes on to say that increasing the pelvic circulation can help to rid the body of some of the bloating associated with PMS. Try to exercise for 20 to 30 minutes at least three times a week. If you are too fatigued to exercise during the actual PMS period, don't. Doing so the rest of the month should help in itself.

Talk it over. Try to explain to your loved ones and close friends the reason for your erratic behavior. "One of the biggest stresses on a woman during this time is family. And it's not only the stress of feeling bad when she flies off the handle at someone, but also of having to apologize for her behavior later on," says Zimmer. He recommends enlisting the aid of your family and close friends by asking them to understand what the problem is and to realize that when you lash out at them you are not as in control as you would like to be. "If your child is really acting out and yelling at you for something during your PMS time, you might remind him that this is not the best time for him to be getting you angry. Hopefully, he'll see this as his cue to go outside and play," Zimmer explains. "You have to walk a fine line, though, and not begin using PMS as an excuse to be nasty to people," he adds.

If the emotional symptoms are causing problems in your relationships, consider getting some counseling from a mental-health professional.

STOMACH UPSET
23 Ways to Tame Your Tummy

If your tummy is bothering you, play detective with your symptoms. It's alimentary, my dear Watson.

First question: How long has this been going on? Chronic, long-term stomach upset is something you should be discussing with your doctor. But if your temperamental tummy is something that hit you after a big meal or a party, it's likely that it's a temporary discomfort.

"We try to separate out the temporary 'I ate too much pizza' from the long-term," says Sherman Hess, B.S., R.Ph., a pharmacist in Portland, Oregon, who has guided many a gastronomically upset customer to the antacid shelf.

Temporary stomach upset may be due to indigestion or flu. Often, it's the result of something—or the quantity of something—you ate. Here are some tips that can help you.

Try some soda. Soda pop, particularly 7-Up and other non-caffeinated varieties, helps to settle stomachs, says Hess.

Take fruit juice for flu. If you have the flu, with diarrhea and/or vomiting, fruit juice will help resupply the potassium and other nutrients your body has lost.

Don't count on milk. Douglas C. Walta, M.D., a gastroenterologist in Portland, Oregon, says milk often hinders stomachs because some people can't digest it easily. "Milk is probably the biggest contributor to gut upset that I see in the population over 30," he says.

Ease off on coffee. Coffee may irritate the stomach. "It's controversial whether it's the acid or the caffeine or both," says Walta.

WHAT'S IT TO YOU?

"**W**hat you consider indigestion and what I consider indigestion is very variable," says Douglas C. Walta, M.D.

The word can be tagged to a wide range of maladies, some of them simple, some of them serious. Walta says he tells patients to drop the word "indigestion" and to just describe to him their gut feelings. Also, it's helpful to him to know if patients feel better or worse after eating. They may be describing what could be a pre-ulcer disease or a gallbladder problem. In some cases, especially in older individuals, the symptoms may be tied to a cancerous condition.

That's why Walta is concerned about attaching the label "indigestion" to too many symptoms. The rule of thumb is, if the condition persists, see a doctor.

Hold off on the booze. Alcohol also is an irritant to the stomach lining, Walta says.

Lighten up on pepper. Red and black pepper are frequently identified as gastrointestinal irritants, says Kimra Warren, R.D., a registered dietitian at St. Vincent Hospital and Medical Center in Portland, Oregon. Try cutting back to see if your symptoms improve. If they don't, then pepper isn't your problem.

Don't smoke. Walta notes that smoking is often associated with ulcers. Cigarette smoke is a gastrointestinal irritant.

Watch your diet. Do your stomach a favor and eat foods that are easy to digest. David M. Taylor, M.D., a gastroenterologist and assistant professor of medicine at Emory University in Atlanta and the Medical College of Georgia in Augusta, says the stomach has a tough time with fatty, fried foods. "A high-carbohydrate, low-fat, high-bulk diet is the best thing," he says.

Increase fiber gradually. A high-fiber diet is good for your health, but don't go too high too fast. A gradual change of diet, with a slow but continual addition of fiber, will help to offset tolerance problems.

Choose veggies carefully. You may love broccoli, but if you have a problem with gas, perhaps you should cut back, suggests Warren. Too much of certain gassy vegetables, namely broccoli, cauliflower, and brussels sprouts, can be a problem.

Limit problematic fruits. Some people get tummy problems from eating apples and melon. Pay attention to whether your stomach upset followed eating one of these.

Worry about the quantity, not quality. Walta says it's a myth that hot, spicy foods create stomach problems. So go ahead and eat spicy food. Just don't overload your stomach.

Cook gasless beans. Warren says if you throw out the water in which you've soaked the beans overnight, and cook them in fresh water, you'll significantly decrease their gas-causing potential.

Think about your diet. Problem foods can be very individualistic. Identify the foods that bother your stomach, then avoid them.

Exercise your body. "Exercise is very helpful," says Taylor. Even a brief walk, particularly after meals, may aid in digestion and help you feel better.

Drink plenty of water. Nutritionists recommend six to eight glasses of water a day to help with digestion.

Avoid laxatives. If you have constipation, it's better to avoid laxatives, says Taylor. Instead, go the more natural route and take bran or a commercial bulking agent such as Metamucil.

Lay off the aspirin. Aspirin and nonsteroidal anti-inflammatory drugs, such as ibuprofen, can actually create ulcers. "What causes ulcers to bleed is aspirin," says Walta. If you have a sensitive stomach but you need pain relief, try acetaminophen or enteric-coated aspirin.

Take an antacid. Antacids are very effective in soothing stomachs, but they can have side effects. For example, magnesium-based antacids can cause diarrhea, while calcium-based antacids can cause constipation. Antacids with aluminum hydroxide also can cause constipation.

Switch brands. Sometimes, a different brand of antacid may prove to be more effective.

Don't take an antacid too long. Side effects from the use of an antacid usually don't appear unless a person has taken the medication for several days. But if the stomach problem has persisted that long, it's time to consult a doctor.

Try an antacid in tablet form. Hess suggests taking an antacid in tablet form because the dose is lower than in liquid preparations and therefore may not contribute to constipation or diarrhea.

Relax. After disease is ruled out as the cause of stomach discomfort, the underlying culprit often turns out to be stress. Stress frequently translates into physical problems. Along the gastrointestinal tract, these problems can include indigestion, irritable bowel syndrome, constipation, and diarrhea.

The cure: Unwind. Relax. Enjoy yourself. Taylor says he recommends "hobbies, running or tennis or hiking or karate, or communing with nature, or sex, or whatever" to patients whose stomach troubles seem to be stress related. He says one of the most effective prescriptions is to take a trip. "They come back and say, 'Gee, doc, it's remarkable. I went away skiing and now I don't have any trouble.'"

TOOTHACHE

9 Ways to Ease the Pain

"For there was never yet philosopher that could endure the toothache patiently." Shakespeare was right. The toothache isn't easy to endure. The good news: With improved dental care and regular checkups, the excruciating pain of a toothache is not as common as it once was. But when pain does occur in the mouth, it's an important signal that you should not ignore—even if it goes away on its own.

Tooth pain is varied. Perhaps most common is the minor pain caused by sensitive teeth. You eat or drink something hot, cold, or sweet and feel a momentary twinge. Some people suffer achy teeth because of sinus problems; that's probably

TOOTHACHE MYTHS

Don't fall for these myths—you could end up causing more damage by believing in them.

Put an aspirin on the tooth. If you want to use aspirin to help relieve the pain of a toothache, swallow it with a glass of water. Do not place it on the tooth or surrounding gum. "That's a fallacy," says Joseph Tenca, D.D.S., M.A. "Aspirin does not work locally." What's worse, you may end up with a severe burn from the aspirin on your gum or cheek that can take four to five days to heal. "You're only adding to your problems," he says.

A toothache means you'll lose the tooth. Not so anymore. "Just because you have a bad toothache doesn't mean the tooth will have to be extracted," reassures Tenca. Root-canal therapy can save an abscessed tooth or one with damaged pulp. Root-canal therapy involves making a small opening in the tooth, removing the pulp in the root canal (that's where the name of the procedure comes from), filling the canal with a material called gutta percha, and then, usually, crowning the tooth. Sometimes, tiny metal posts are placed in the canal to help strengthen the tooth.

If the pain disappears, the problem's gone. "You don't have that kind of pain for no reason," says Alan H. Gluskin, D.D.S. He points out that coronary problems can cause pain in the lower jaw, while mouth pain can be referred to the ears, neck, or even shoulder. "Don't ever ignore pain in the head and neck."

the case if you notice that the pain is limited to your upper teeth and that several teeth are affected at one time. Recent dental work can cause a tooth to be sensitive to temperature changes for a few weeks.

But some types of pain deserve immediate attention from your dentist. If you feel a sharp pain when you bite down, for instance, you may have a cavity, a loose filling, a cracked tooth, or damaged pulp (that's the inner core of the tooth that contains the blood vessels and nerves). Pain that sticks around for more than 30 minutes after eating hot or cold foods can also indicate pulp damage, either from a deep cavity or a blow to the tooth. And the stereotypical toothache with constant and severe pain, swelling, and sensitivity is definitely a sign of trouble. "If the pain wakes you up at night, it's serious," says Joseph Tenca, D.D.S., M.A., past president of the

WHEN PULP GOES BAD

Most of us don't think of our teeth as being alive, but they are. Each tooth contains what's called the pulp, composed of nourishing blood vessels and nerves.

If that pulp is damaged or exposed, the nerves can die, and the tooth can become infected, or abscessed. What can cause this? A deep cavity, a cracked tooth, or a hard blow to the tooth (from biting down on a popcorn kernel, for example).

"Once the pulp has been damaged or exposed, it can't repair itself," says Roland C. Duell, D.D.S., M.S. "It will need treatment." That's why you need to pay attention to any pain you experience from your teeth.

American Association of Endodontists and professor and chairman of the Department of Endodontics at Tufts University School of Dental Medicine in Boston. You could have an abscessed tooth; that means the pulp of the tooth has died, resulting in an infection that can spread to the gum and bone.

Pain associated with the pulp of the tooth is kind of tricky. It can let you know that damage has occurred. "But the degeneration of the nerves (in the pulp) can be very rapid," points out Alan H. Gluskin, D.D.S., associate professor and chairperson of the Department of Endodontics at the University of the Pacific School of Dentistry in San Francisco. "They can die within a 12-hour period." So the pain disappears. But then the tooth hurts again as the dead tissue becomes infected, or abscessed.

That's why putting off dental attention for a toothache can mean bad news. But if it's 3:00 in the morning or the middle of Sunday afternoon, you can take some temporary measures to deal with the pain until you can get into the dental office:

Take two aspirin . . . or acetaminophen or ibuprofen, "whatever over-the-counter analgesic you use to relieve your headaches," says Tenca. Roland C. Duell, D.D.S., M.S., professor of endodontics with the Department of Oral Health Practice at the University of Kentucky College of Dentistry in Lexington, points out that ibuprofen is best at relieving inflammation, which may accompany a toothache.

Apply oil of cloves. You can pick this up at the pharmacy. Follow the directions for use, and be sure to put it only on the tooth and NOT on the gum. Otherwise, your burning gums may distract you from your toothache. And remember, oil of cloves won't cure the toothache; it just numbs the nerve.

Cool the swelling. Put a cold compress on the outside of your cheek if you've got swelling from the toothache.

Chill the pain. Holding an ice cube or cold water in the mouth may relieve the pain, says Tenca. But if you find that it simply aggravates your sensitive tooth, skip it.

Keep your head up. Elevating your head can decrease the pressure in the area, says Duell.

Rinse. You can't really rinse away the pain, but you can rinse with warm water to remove any food debris. Tenca suggests using one teaspoon of salt in a glass of warm water.

Floss. No, it's not a cure, but flossing is another way to remove any food debris that could be trapped. The rubber tip on your toothbrush or a toothpick (if used with caution) can help dislodge any stuck food. "Sometimes, food can get lodged in the gum, and the pain mimics that caused by pulpal problems," says Tenca.

Be careful with the hot, the cold, and the sweet. These foods and beverages may aggravate an already sore and sensitive situation.

Plug it. If the tooth feels sensitive to air, cover it with gauze or even sugarless chewing gum until you can get to the dentist.

VARICOSE VEINS

16 Coping Techniques

The circulatory system could be compared to a big city's freeways, where the bumper-to-bumper cars, in this case the frenetic blood cells, are delivering oxygen and nutrients to every part of the body. The pumping heart maintains the pulse of the "traffic" by pushing the blood cells on their way through the arteries.

On the cells' return trip to the heart and lungs, the veins have a harder time of it. For one thing, the pressure caused by the pumping heart is decreased. For another, the veins below the heart, in the legs and torso, must work against gravity, as the blood makes its way up from the feet. So these vessels depend more on the leg muscles to help pump the blood back to the heart. The veins also contain valves to help keep the blood moving along. The valves work like locks in a canal. As blood flows through a valve, its "doors" slam shut so the blood can't go backward.

When any one of these valves fail, blood can seep back and begin to pool, often in the lower legs. The extra pressure of the increased volume of pooling blood can, over time, cause subsequent valves to fail. Then the vein's walls begin to bulge and become misshapen. At this point, the vein may show through the skin surface, looking knotty and gnarled, blue and bumpy.

It's estimated that 25 percent of all women and 10 percent of all men are affected by varicose veins. Fortunately, there are ways to prevent or, at the very least, postpone, their development and decrease their severity. Here's how:

Check your family tree. "The tendency to develop varicose veins can run in families," says Hugh Gelabert, M.D., assistant professor of surgery in the Section of Vascular Surgery at the University of California at Los Angeles School of Medicine. The reason for this is unknown. Some experts believe there is a weakness in the gene that governs the development of the veins. This may lead to defects in the structure of valves and veins or, in some people, a decrease in the number of valves in the veins, causing the few that are there to get overloaded in their duties. If you do find a history of varicose veins in your family, the sooner you follow preventative measures the better.

Get moving. "Exercise works by keeping the veins empty of pooling blood," says Gelabert. "Every time a muscle contracts in the buttocks, thighs, or lower legs, blood is helped on its way back to the heart." However, it's hard

SPIDER VEINS: "COUSIN" TO VARICOSE VEINS

Eighty percent of varicose-vein sufferers will also develop spider veins, says Luis Navarro, M.D. And half of all spider-vein sufferers also have varicose veins. But unlike knotty varicose veins, spider veins are thin and weblike in appearance (thus the name) and most often show up on the legs, neck, and face. These veins are actually dilated blood vessels that appear no thicker than a thread or hair. Except for their link to pregnancy and hormones (see "Advice for Moms-to-Be" on page 199), no one knows for sure why they crop up. Because the cause hasn't been pinpointed, the veins can't be prevented. But, they rarely cause problems—perhaps only a little itching now and again.

to say if exercise will only postpone, or if it can prevent, varicose veins. "If there's a strong family history of the condition present, then exercise will probably only postpone the condition," says Gelabert. To get your legs moving, almost any exercise that involves the legs will do, from aerobics to strengthening to spot-toning activities, say the experts. Ride a bike, take an aerobics class, go for a walk or a run, use the stair machine in the gym—these are all good exercises for the legs. Spot-toning exercises, such as leg raises, that specifically build up the muscles in the buttocks, thighs, and lower legs are also recommended.

Lose weight. Obesity "puts a strain on every part of the body," explains Luis Navarro, M.D., founder and director of the Vein Treatment Center in New York and author of *No More Varicose Veins*. "Furthermore, people who are overweight tend to be more immobile and get less exercise." As a result, overweight people usually have muscles that can't as efficiently help the veins pump their blood back to the heart. In addition, an overweight person's blood vessels carry more blood than a thinner person's, so the strain is greater on the vessels themselves.

Eat a balanced diet. Besides helping you to maintain proper weight, a balanced diet can give you nutrients that may actually help prevent varicose veins. Protein and vitamin C are both components of collagen, part of the tissue in the veins and valves. If the collagen is in good shape, the tissues may not fall apart as readily. However, "diet will not reverse a case of varicose veins," says Frank J. Veith, M.D., professor of surgery and chief of Vascular Surgical Services at Montefiore Medical Center–Albert Einstein College of Medicine in New York.

Take a break from standing. "When you're upright, the feet are the furthest possible distance away from the heart, so the blood has far to go, against gravity no less, to get back to the heart," says Gelabert. As a result, the blood can have a tendency to pool in the lower legs, leading to the development of varicose veins.

But don't sit too long, either. Some experts theorize that even sitting can contribute to varicose veins. "They believe since the knees and groin are bent while sitting, the blood flow has a difficult course back to the heart," says Navarro. So it's very important on a long car or plane ride or during a day of sitting at the office that you get up and stretch your legs once in a while. Navarro suggests this rejuvenator: Stand on your toes and flex the heel up and down ten times.

Get support from your stockings. Support panty hose are better than regular hosiery for helping to control the development of varicose veins. Better yet are the support stockings available by prescription. These stockings help by keeping the veins in the legs from bulging, and as a result, keeping fluids from collecting in the legs. How do they work? They apply more pressure to the lower legs than to the thigh area. Since more pressure is exerted on the lower legs, blood is more readily pushed up toward the heart. The stockings' compression on the legs is measured in millimeters of mercury, called mm Hg, and ranges from 20 mm Hg for milder cases to 60 mm Hg for severe varicosity. (In comparison, support panty hose from a department store have a strength of 14 mm Hg to 17 mm Hg.) The prescription stockings also come in a variety of lengths: below the knee, midthigh, full thigh, and waist high. The lower-strength stockings are some-

ADVICE FOR MOMS-TO-BE

Pregnancy can also lead to the development of varicose veins and spider veins. Surging hormones weaken collagen and connective tissues in the pelvis in preparation for giving birth. Unfortunately, as a side effect, the hormones may also weaken the collagen found in the veins and valves of the body. These weakened tissues have a more difficult time standing up to the increased blood volume that comes with carrying a baby. In addition, the weight of the fetus itself may play a role in the development of varicose veins and spider veins in the legs, says Hugh Gelabert, M.D. Elevating the legs whenever possible can be helpful, and compression stockings in the 20 mm Hg to 30 mm Hg range may be prescribed. The good news is that for many women, the swollen veins subside after the baby is born.

times recommended for pregnant women (see "Advice for Moms-to-Be"). Since the stockings are only available in a few colors, some women prefer to wear them under pants. The downside: The stockings have a tendency to feel hot.

Slip into spandex pants. Like store-bought support panty hose, this type of stretch pant applies pressure to the legs, says Gelabert.

Cover up the blues. If you've stopped wearing shorts or going to the beach because you're embarrassed about your varicose veins, make them "disappear." There are products specially made to cover the blue vein lines that are causing you to take cover. Available in a variety of shades to match your skin, the cream is applied by hand and blended. Leg Magic by Covermark Cosmetics is waterproof and even has a sun protection factor (SPF) of 16 to protect your legs from the sun's harmful rays. Wearing stockings over the cover-up won't make it fade or rub off, and you can even go for a swim, says Richard Ottaviano, president of Covermark Cosmetics in Moonachie, New Jersey. While these types of products obviously won't fix the veins, they may make you feel better about yourself.

CLOTS: BE CAREFUL!

Though thankfully rare, clots can form in varicose veins. Thrombophlebitis, the inflammation of a vein caused by a clot, can be potentially dangerous if the clot begins to travel through the veins. The traveling clot, then called an embolism, can end up blocking part of the blood flow in the heart or lungs, possibly resulting in a pulmonary (lung) embolism or in heart failure.

If the clot forms in what's called the superficial venous system, "you may see localized redness at the site, as well as tenderness and pain," says Alan M. Dietzek, M.D. If the clot forms in what's known as the deep venous system, you won't be able to see the clot, but you may have swelling and tenderness in all or part of either leg, he says. If you experience any of these symptoms, see your doctor.

Some of the best measures to help prevent clotting: Keep active; maintain a desirable weight; and take breaks from sitting, especially on long car and plane rides and during long hours of sitting at work.

Consider the effects of estrogen. The hormone is generally believed to have a detrimental effect on the collagen and connective tissue of the veins. And "while the Pill probably does not have a direct correlation to varicose veins, it may have an indirect one," says Gelabert. "The Pill may lead to the development of embolisms, or clots in the blood, which can interfere with blood flow" (see "Clots: Be Careful!").

Prop up your legs. Elevating the legs is good, but raising them above your heart is even better. By doing this, you're working with gravity to help get the blood out of the ankles and back to the heart. "This is the oldest and most successful way to alleviate discomfort and facilitate drainage and reduce swelling," says Gelabert. As a matter of fact, Hippocrates in ancient Greece wrote of its benefits, he notes. Lie down on a couch and put your feet on the back of it. "If you can, elevate the legs for ten minutes every hour," recommends Alan M. Dietzek, M.D., vascular surgeon at North Shore University Hospital in

Manhasset, New York, and assistant professor of surgery at Cornell Medical College in New York.

Flex your feet. "Flexing might help by making the muscles contract, which in turn helps squeeze the blood out of the veins," explains Gelabert. While your legs are elevated, try these three exercises to keep the blood pumping out of your feet and back to your heart:

• The Ankle Pump: Flex your foot up and down as you would when you pump a piano pedal or gas pedal.

• Ankle Circles: Rotate your feet clockwise and counterclockwise.

• Heel Slips: With your knees bent, slide your heels back and forth.

Sleep with elevated feet. For those with chronic swelling in the lower legs, it may help to put a few pillows under your feet while sleeping, says Gelabert.

Wear tennis shoes. If your feet habitually swell, it may be worthwhile to wear tennis shoes or other lace-up shoes that can be loosened to alleviate the pressure.

WEIGHT GAIN

37 Ways to Fight the Battle of the Bulge

At any given moment, 33 to 40 percent of American women and 20 to 24 percent of American men are trying to lose weight. Yet an estimated one-fourth to one-third of Americans are still overweight, which increases their risk for heart disease, high blood pressure, and Type II (noninsulin-dependent) diabetes as well as for gallbladder disease, gout, some types of cancer, and osteoarthritis.

Traditional knowledge says that 3,500 calories equal one pound of weight. Cut the calories or burn more of them than you consume, and you'll drop pounds. That's been the approach for years—but it isn't working. Short-term diets that restrict calories can help you lose, but as much as two-thirds of that weight is generally regained within a year and almost all of it within five years.

Weight loss is more complicated than a simple equation. That was part of the conclusion drawn from a conference sponsored by the National Institutes of Health in the spring of 1992. "Overweight is not a simple disorder of willpower, as sometimes implied, but is a complex disorder of energy metabolism," stated the conference report.

Many diets just don't work for the long haul. If you really want to keep the weight off for the rest of your life, you have to change your lifestyle. "Someday, I hope we'll look back on semistarvation diets the way we currently view such archaic practices as bleeding and purging," says C. Wayne Callaway, M.D., associate clinical professor of medicine at George Washington University in Washington, D.C., and a member of the 1989–1990 Dietary Guidelines Advisory Committee to the U.S. Department of Agriculture. "You have to look at weight loss as a lifetime management issue," says Callaway. "A weight problem is not like having pneumonia where you can take a course of antibiotics and cure it. You have to keep working on your weight."

Dieting becomes a way of life for some people, particularly women, who lose and gain over and over again in a syndrome of "yo-yo" dieting. A 1991 study published in *The New England Journal of Medicine* indicates that you may be shortening your life span if you engage in such practices. And most research has shown that such weight cycling probably makes it easier to regain the weight by messing with your metabolism (the rate at which your body burns calories). "You lose eight pounds of fat and two pounds of muscle the first time," explains Gabe Mirkin, M.D., associate professor at Georgetown University Medical School in Washington, D.C., and author of *The Mirkin Report*, a monthly newsletter on health, fitness, and nutrition. "Then you gain back ten pounds—all of it fat. So you've increased your amount of fat by two pounds," says Mirkin. Ironically, adds Callaway, you've lost muscle mass, and muscle actually helps burn more calories.

How do you lose fat wisely and increase your chances of keeping it off? The experts suggest:

Decide first if you truly need to lose weight. Look at your shape, height, weight, and history of obesity-linked diseases and the history of those factors in your family, suggests Callaway. Then consider when your weight prob-

DO YOU NEED TO LOSE WEIGHT?

Many of us, particularly women, don't care what the various charts say about our height-weight ratios. We're striving for a certain look, and unfortunately, that body image may be impossible for some of us to attain.

How do you know if you need to lose weight? You can check the Metropolitan Life Insurance Company Height and Weight Tables, which were revised in 1983. To determine your risk for weight-related health problems, however, consider the following:

• **Are you at risk for high blood pressure, Type II diabetes, or heart disease?** Your physician can help you with those answers by examining your medical and family history, along with performing certain diagnostic tests.

• **Where's your fat located?** If it's concentrated around your belly, you need to lose. If it's around your hips and thighs but your belly's flat, you can relax a bit. That's because abdominal fat is linked with a higher risk for medical conditions than is fat on the hips and thighs. Divide your waist measurement by your hip measurement to get your waist/hip ratio: .70 to .75 is considered healthy for women and .80 to .90 is considered healthy for men. If you're above that, you need to lose.

• **Calculate your body mass index (BMI).** Divide your weight in pounds by 2.2 to get kilograms and your height in inches by 39.37 to get meters. Your BMI equals weight in kilograms divided by height in meters squared. Normal BMI is considered to be between 19 and 27.

lems began: Have you gained weight recently as the result of a marital separation or is this a gradual pattern since your teens? (See "Do You Need to Lose Weight?")

Analyze your eating and activity patterns. "If you're starving and bingeing, you first have to learn how to eat normally," says Callaway. He's seen numerous patients on low-calorie diets who persist in gaining weight, despite how much they cut down on what they eat. He blames constant dieting and erratic eating habits for reducing their metabolic rates, forcing their bodies into a starvation mode that hoards fat.

Keep a food diary for two weeks. Write down everything you eat, when you eat it, and how you're feeling at the time—bored, angry, or hungry, for example. "A food diary can be illuminating to a lot of people," points out Barbara Deskins, Ph.D., R.D., associate professor of clinical dietetics and nutrition at the University of Pittsburgh. "They don't realize they eat automatically." If you decide to visit a registered dietitian for assistance, take your food diary along.

Make a plan. Once you decide you're ready to change your lifestyle to reach a desirable weight, you'll have to figure out how to do that. Most experts recommend learning to make nutritionally sound food choices, eating an adequate amount of food each day, and increasing your physical activity. You may find the advice of your family physician, a registered dietitian, or an exercise physiologist helpful. (Callaway cautions, however, that you should make sure that the dietitian sticks to nutritional counseling and the exercise physiologist to exercise.) Some university medical centers and hospitals are adopting a multidisciplinary team to handle weight loss; a registered dietitian, a physician, an exercise physiologist, and a behavioral psychologist join forces.

If you decide to go it alone, however, the tips that follow can help.

Don't plan to lose too much too soon. Rapid weight loss generally means a rapid weight gain down the road, says Callaway. Don't try to lose more than half a pound a week.

Pick a good time. "Don't decide to start this the week before your wedding or right after you lose your job," says Deskins. "You don't want to choose a period of high stress only to add additional stress."

Don't try to change everything at once. "It's unrealistic to think that tomorrow you'll completely redo your food habits in some 180-degree shift," says Deskins. Make changes gradually.

Start with damage control. If you're the family food shopper, you can handle this one yourself. Or discuss it with the person who does the grocery shopping. It's pretty simple advice: If you don't have potato chips or chocolate around, you're not as likely to indulge in these high-calo-

DIETING AND PREGNANCY DON'T MIX

One time not to diet, say the experts: at the beginning of your pregnancy, even if you are overweight. "If you weigh 400 pounds, you still need to gain 20 pounds during pregnancy," says Gabe Mirkin, M.D. "It's important to eat regularly and not to skip meals," adds Barbara Deskins, Ph.D., R.D. Skipping meals can cause the body to break down its fat reserves, which create certain by-products known as ketones that may harm the fetus.

rie snacks. Instead, keep low-calorie snacks and foods on hand—raw vegetables or rice cakes, whatever works. The same thing goes in terms of the food that gets cooked for meals. Overweight tends to run in families, and part of that is due to shared eating habits, says John H. Renner, M.D., president of the Consumer Health Information Research Institute in Kansas City, Missouri, and member of the Board of Directors of the National Council Against Health Fraud.

Measure your foods. Doing this tedious chore for a few days can help train your eye to recognize portion sizes, says Johanna Dwyer, D.Sc., R.D., professor at Tufts University School of Nutrition and Tufts University Medical School and director of the Frances Stern Nutrition Center at New England Medical Center Hospitals, all in Boston.

Don't count calories. Opinions differ on this one, but most experts suggest changing the way you eat, rather than allotting yourself only so many calories a day.

Cut out the alcohol. You could say a martini is "empty calories"—it has no nutritional benefits. Callaway points out that alcohol may encourage fat distribution around the waist. The average American gets ten percent of calories from alcohol, says Deskins, so abstinence for some could mean a substantial drop in calories. "Some people can lose weight just by giving up beer," says Renner.

Eat breakfast. And lunch. And dinner. Callaway explains that skipping meals leads to binge eating. It's the body's attempt to make up for lack of food intake as it goes into starvation mode. He says if you get one-fourth of your calories at each meal, you'll lose the urge to snack as well.

Make sure you eat enough. That's music to any dieter's ears, but Callaway is concerned that starvation diets lead to bingeing and lowered metabolism.

Don't make a lapse a collapse. Just because you fail one day and pig out on the wrong foods doesn't mean you should give up for good, says Dwyer. Pick yourself up, dust yourself off, and start over again the next day.

Get your nutrients. You need two servings a day of meat, fish, poultry, or meat substitutes like eggs, legumes, or nuts; two servings of dairy products (three for children and four for teenagers); four servings of fruits and vegetables; and four servings of breads, cereals, pastas, and other grains.

Cut the fat. Fat is where it's at if you want to target one enemy of your waistline. And cutting out high-fat foods can benefit much more than your figure—you'll lower your risk for heart disease and some cancers. Fat is nature's way of crowding a lot of calories—or energy—into food. A gram of fat (one-fourth of a teaspoon) contains nine calories, while a gram of protein or carbohydrate has four.

How much fat is too much? The average American is consuming about 37 percent of calories from fat these days, down from 40 percent a few years ago, says Deskins. The American Heart Association recommends that no more than 30 percent of your calories come from fat, while Mirkin says if you also want to really reduce cholesterol, you'll have to go much lower than that.

High-fat foods can fool you, too. "They're small in amount but high in calories," says Dwyer. Follow these pointers to cut the fat:

• Switch to reduced-fat or nonfat salad dressing.

• Buy nonstick pans and use a tiny amount of oil or nonstick spray.

• Eat less meat and cheese; both can be high in fat.

• Buy lean cuts of meat and trim the fat before cooking. Remove the skin from poultry.

• Don't fry. Instead, roast, bake, broil, or simmer meat, poultry, and fish.

• Choose low-fat dairy products, such as skim milk.

EMPTY PROMISES

Weight loss is big business in this country, with Americans spending more than $30 billion a year on various products and programs. It's an area ripe for quacks and frauds, who promise more than they can possibly deliver. In fact, the Federal Trade Commission has investigated the advertising and marketing claims of a number of diet products and programs over the last two years. Here's what John H. Renner, M.D., says to watch out for:

- Words like "melt away," "no effort," "painless," "no exercise"
- Plans or programs that promise excessive weight loss, such as a pound a day
- Programs that depend on artificial food or pills
- Claims that a food, such as grapefruit, possesses magical properties to get rid of excess weight
- Diets or gadgets that claim to cause weight loss from just one part of the body, such as the buttocks or chin
- Multilevel marketing plans that involve purchasing and selling products to people you know ("You shouldn't be buying your weight-loss products from your Sunday-school teacher," Renner points out.)

- Fill up your plate with vegetables, fruits, and grains, and don't drown them in butter.
- Experiment with spices; use them to add flavor to your foods.
- Avoid nondairy creamers and toppings, which often contain high amounts of saturated fats from palm or coconut oils.

Exercise. Even nutritionists agree: Exercise appears to be the key in losing weight. "The leanest people in this country eat the most food, but they're the most active," says Callaway.

Obviously, exercise burns calories. But according to some researchers, it may also increase your metabolism, possibly for as long as 18 hours after you've worked out, says Mirkin. So you end up burning more calories, even after your workout.

The effects of adding exercise to your life will vary depending on how active you already are. If you're a couch

FAT KIDS

It's very likely that television has contributed to the creation of a generation of fat kids. Obesity is on the increase among children.

Although following the weight-control guidelines for adults can certainly help, you may want some advice specifically targeted to kids:

Teach them how to select foods. "If you can't change where they eat, then teach them to make more healthy choices," says Ted Williams, M.D., a pediatrician in private practice in Dothan, Alabama, and a media spokesperson for the American Academy of Pediatrics. Encourage them to choose pizza with vegetable toppings instead of meat toppings, get a cheeseburger made with ground turkey, use low-fat cheese, pick a whole-grain bun over white bread, get pasta instead of french fries, and so on.

Set a good example. Don't just tell them what to do, show them by adopting the same healthy habits.

Give them low-fat milk. Once your children are over the age of two years, encourage them to drink low-fat milk. Williams says that children who consume one to one-and-a-half quarts of whole milk a day are getting a large amount of saturated fat in their diet.

Kick kids out of the house. Get them to exercise—it doesn't have to be a structured program. Encourage them to play; they'll burn off calories and excess weight that way, whether they're biking or at the playground.

Take the children with you while you exercise. Make sure you're getting some exercise on a regular basis. Walking's one way. "Take the kids with you," Williams suggests.

Don't become overzealous. Some parents attempt to put their children on a low-fat diet too early in life. Children under the age of two years actually need a certain amount of fat in their diet for the proper development of the nervous system, according to Williams.

potato, the benefits you'll get from brisk walking may surprise you. If you're already exercising occasionally, you may need more aggressive exercise like running or cycling.

Callaway stresses the need to first change your eating patterns before working on adding physical activity to your life. Once you feel comfortable with those changes, concentrate on the physical. Get help from your local YMCA or hire a personal trainer if you need advice.

Use these tricks to get your body moving:

• Take the stairs instead of the elevator.

• Park farther away.

• Walk instead of riding or driving.

• Take several short walks if you can't fit one 30-minute workout into your schedule.

If you need more vigorous excerise:

• Cross-train. Because intense exercise can break down muscle tissue, you want to give those muscles 48 hours to replace themselves between workouts, says Mirkin. You can take a day off, of course, or you can alternate exercises that work different muscle groups: Use a rowing machine on Monday and run on Tuesday, for example.

• Alternate hard and easy. You can try this practice to avoid injury as well. Work out hard one day, easy the next: Run, then walk, for example. "Sixty-five percent of the people who take up running or aerobics quit within six weeks because of injury," Mirkin says. Alternating activities and intensity can help keep you from dropping out of exercise.

• Try strength training as well. "Lean body mass, or muscle, burns more calories," says Callaway. Aerobic exercise isn't the only way to lose weight. By including some resistance training in your program, you'll create more muscle mass.

YEAST INFECTIONS

12 Strategies to Beat Them

Most women are bothered at one time or another by the itching, burning, pain, and discharge that comes with a vaginal infection. Yeast infections can be caused by a number of organisms, many of which inhabit the healthy vagina. One of the most common causes of vaginitis is the fungus *Candida albicans*.

HELLO, DOCTOR?

While mild cases of yeast infection can be effectively treated at home, Sadja Greenwood, M.D., says it's important to see a physician if:

• You have abdominal pain.

• You have recurrent or significant amounts of bloody discharge between periods.

• The discharge gets worse or persists for two weeks or more despite treatment.

• You may have been exposed to a sexually transmitted disease.

• You have recurrent yeast infections. You may have diabetes or a prediabetic condition that is contributing to your yeast infections.

• Your discharge is thin, foamy, and grey or yellowish green in color.

"Yeast infections are characterized by itching, caked discharge that smells like baking bread, and reddening of the labia and sometimes upper thighs," says Felicia Stewart, M.D., a gynecologist in Sacramento, California.

Yeast infections, especially recurrent ones, are a signal that your body is out of balance. *Candida* normally grows in a healthy vagina, but the slightly acid pH environment keeps *Candida* and other microorganisms from multiplying rapidly enough to cause infection. However, a variety of factors can make the body go "tilt" and alter the vaginal pH enough to allow one or more microorganisms to grow unchecked. The itching, burning, pain, and discharge are caused by the waste products of rapidly multiplying *Candida* (or other) organisms.

There are plenty of things that can throw your body out of balance. Many women find they are more vulnerable to yeast infection under these conditions:

• **Pregnancy.** The hormonal changes associated with pregnancy alter the vaginal pH and increase carbohydrate (glycogen) production, which provides food for infectious organisms.

• **Menstruation.** Some women report more yeast flare-ups just before or just after their menstrual period.

• **Antibiotics.** *Candida* live in the healthy vagina in balance with other microorganisms, especially lactobacilli. Tetracycline and other antibiotics kill the vagina's lactobacilli and allow *Candida* to multiply, says Sadja Greenwood, M.D., assistant clinical professor in the Department of Obstetrics, Gynecology, and Reproductive Sciences at the University of California at San Francisco. Some antibiotics, especially tetracycline, also appear to stimulate the growth of yeast organisms.

• **Diabetes or a high-sugar diet.** High blood sugar caused by diabetes or by a high-sugar diet can change vaginal pH and contribute to yeast infections. "Some women," says Stewart, "drink lots of fruit juice to prevent bladder infections. But fruit juice contains so much sugar, it may promote yeast infections."

• **Stressful times.** Doctors don't fully understand the stress/yeast connection, but many women report an increase in yeast infections during times of high stress.

While yeast infections can often be treated successfully at home, be sure yeast is the culprit. Other organisms, which require medical treatment, may be causing your symptoms. If the discharge is foul-smelling, yellowish, and frothy, you may be infected by one-celled protozoans called *trichomonas* or "trick." If you have a heavy discharge without much irritation and notice a fishy odor, particularly after intercourse, your symptoms may be caused by a bacterial infection doctors call "bacterial vaginosis." Bacterial infections are the most common cause of vaginitis. Both of these infections require treatment with prescription medication. In addition, symptoms similar to those of vaginitis may be caused by sexually transmitted diseases such as gonorrhea or chlamydia. *It's important to have your vaginal symptoms evaluated by a physician to ensure proper treatment.*

Many women who suffer from recurrent yeast infections have had their symptoms diagnosed by a doctor and know all too well the signs and symptoms of a yeast flare-up. If you're sure your vaginitis is caused by a yeast infection, try these home remedies:

Use a vinegar douche. At the first sign of infection, try douching with a mild vinegar or yogurt douche, suggests Stewart. For a vinegar douche, use one to three tablespoons of white vinegar to one quart of warm water; for a yogurt douche, make a dilute mixture of plain yogurt and warm water (see "Self-Care Douche" on page 213).

Bring on the boric. Several studies have shown boric acid to be a safe, inexpensive, and effective yeast remedy. Amanda Clark, M.D., assistant professor of obstetrics and gynecology at Oregon Health Sciences University in Portland, suggests using boric-acid capsules as a suppository. "You can't buy the capsules already made up," she says. "Buy size 'O' gelatin capsules and fill them with boric acid. Then insert one per day vaginally for seven days." (Check with your pharmacist for the gelatin capsules and boric acid.)

Boric acid hasn't been studied among pregnant women. If you're pregnant, Clark says to skip the boric acid. Instead, talk with your physician about other treatment options.

Use an over-the-counter antifungal cream. Stewart says both miconazole (Monistat) and clotrimazole (Gyne-Lotrimin) are effective in treating yeast infections. They've recently become available in pharmacies without prescription. Use the suppositories nightly for three days or the cream once daily for one week. Don't stop using the medication when your symptoms subside. Use it for the full course. If recurrent yeast infections are a problem, try using one of these antifungal creams a few days before and/or after your menstrual period.

Try yogurt tabs. "Some women find relief using Lactinex (lactobacillus) tablets vaginally once or twice a day and douching with vinegar twice a day for two days," says Greenwood.

Wash out the secretions. The organisms that cause yeast infection produce secretions that are irritating to the genital tissues, says Clark. The nerve endings that sense the presence of the yeast are located at the vaginal opening. Although you may have an infection inside the vagina, you can often get symptomatic relief, she says, by simply washing away the secretions with water or with a douche.

Stay dry and loose. Yeast organisms like warm, moist conditions, with little or no oxygen. In order to deny them the perfect growing medium, be careful to dry your vagi-

SELF-CARE DOUCHE

Routine douching isn't a good idea if you don't have vaginal symptoms. However, for women with yeast-infection symptoms, a mild vinegar douche can help restore the vagina's normal pH (which is about 4.5). Douching with yogurt that contains live lactobacillus or acidophilus bacteria may help restore the friendly microorganisms lost during infection or because of antibiotic use. For the best douche results, follow these easy steps:

1. Prepare the douche solution as outlined in the first remedy.

2. Make sure the container, tube, and irrigation nozzle are very clean. If not, clean them with a good antiseptic solution.

3. Lie in the tub with a folded towel under your buttocks and with your legs parted.

4. Suspend the container 12 to 18 inches above the hips.

5. Insert the nozzle into the vagina with a gentle rotating motion until it encounters resistance (two to four inches).

6. Allow the solution to flow in slowly. Use your fingers to close the vaginal lips until a little pressure builds up inside. This allows the solution to reach the entire internal surface. An effective douche should take ten minutes or so.

nal area thoroughly after bathing or showering. Avoid wearing tight, restrictive clothing that can hold in heat and moisture, and avoid lounging around in a wet bathing suit for long periods of time. Opt for loose clothing and "breathable" cotton underwear and, if you must wear nylons, wear the type that has a cotton-lined panty or crotch.

Avoid harsh soaps, "feminine hygiene" sprays, and perfumed products. "Harsh soaps and hygiene sprays irritate the vagina and throw off its natural balance," says Susan Woodruff, B.S.N., childbirth and parenting education coordinator for Tuality Community Hospital in Hillsboro, Oregon. "Perfumed products contain alcohol that is drying to the tissues and hundreds of other chemicals that can cause irritation."

Rethink your contraception. Women who take birth control pills or use contraceptive sponges appear to be at greater risk for developing yeast infections. While re-

DOUCHE DANGER

The ads for douches admonish women to "feel fresh." And some women erroneously believe that douching after intercourse will prevent pregnancy (it doesn't). But new evidence shows that routine douching may be too much of a good thing and may actually do more harm than good.

Routine douching has been associated with an increased risk of pelvic inflammatory disease," says Felicia Stewart, M.D. "I don't recommend it."

Pelvic inflammatory disease, or PID, is an infection of the uterus, fallopian tubes, or ovaries. It can cause scarring of the fallopian tubes and result in infertility. If the infection spreads to the circulatory system, it can cause death.

According to a 1990 study in *The Journal of the American Medical Association,* women who douched three or more times per month were three-and-a-half times more likely to have PID than women who douched less than once a month.

The symptoms of PID include fever, chills, lower abdominal pain or tenderness, back pain, spotting, pain during or after intercourse, and puslike vaginal discharge. In most cases, a woman does not show all of the symptoms listed. If you have any PID symptoms, consult a physician immediately.

Not only has routine douching been associated with an increased risk of PID, some researchers believe it may increase a woman's risk of developing cervical cancer. A study that appeared in *The American Journal of Epidemiology* showed that women who douched more than once a week were nearly five times as likely to develop cervical cancer as women who douched less often. The researchers suspect that vaginal secretions and normal vaginal bacteria may somehow protect the pelvic area and that routine douching may invite microbes that trigger cancer.

The message is clear: While an occasional douche during an infection might be a good idea, don't make a habit of douching.

searchers haven't established a cause-and-effect relationship between the Pill and yeast, some studies have shown that oral contraceptives increase the glycogen in the vagina (which provides more food for yeast reproduction).

Contraceptive sponges seem to be a yeast culprit, too. "We don't know exactly why contraceptive sponges increase yeast infections," says Stewart, "but we know they alter the vagina's normal ecology." If recurrent yeast infections are a problem for you, Stewart suggests considering an alternative birth control method like condoms, a diaphragm, a cervical cap, or an intrauterine device (IUD).

Have both partners treated. Sexual partners can play "Ping-Pong" with yeast infections by passing the infection back and forth unless both partners are treated. Often, men harbor yeast organisms, especially in the foreskin of an uncircumcised penis, but show no symptoms. When one partner is treated, the other should be treated to avoid reinfection, advises Woodruff.

Wash up and use condoms. Women with yeast infections should ask their lovers to wash up extra carefully before lovemaking. Couples who make love before the infection is completely cured should use condoms during intercourse.

Avoid routine douching. "The American culture is into cleansing," says Woodruff. "But the vagina doesn't need to be cleaned. It does that naturally. Routine douching upsets the vaginal pH and can actually cause yeast infections" (see "Douche Danger").

Practice good hygiene. While yeast is usually passed between sexual partners, Woodruff says it can also be passed to others like children through activities such as shared baths. To ensure you're not passing yeast, she recommends not bathing or sharing towels with your children, washing your hands frequently with soap and water, and washing your clothing in hot water. "The hot water in your washing machine should kill the yeast organisms present in your clothes," says Woodruff. "But if you're really worried about it, toss a cup of white vinegar into your rinse water."

INDEX

INDEX

Flu, 112-116, 189
    analgesic use during, 107-108
    intestinal, 91
    myths, 116
    at-risk populations, 114
    shots, 114
    symptoms, 112-113
    treatment, 113-116
Fluids
    balance of, 93
    in bladder infection, 37
    in common cold, 57
    and constipation, 62, 63
    and hemorrhoids, 131
    intake in colds, 57
    loss of, 107
    retention of, 45, 187
    in stomach upset, 189, 191
Fluoride, 182
Flushes, 161
Food
    allergies, 18
    bland, 95
    and fever, 107
    and headaches, 122-123
    and heartburn, 127
    and hemorrhoids, 130
    in incontinence, 153
    intolerance, 18
    poisoning, 91
Food and Drug Administration,
    70
Formaldehyde, 78, 80
Framingham Heart Study, 136, 143
Fructose, 86

G

Gallbladder, 190
Gangrene, 87, 88
Gargling, common cold and, 59
Gas. *See* Flatulence.
Gastroenteritis, 91, 116
Genes. *See* Heredity.
Giardia, 92
Ginseng, 47
Glands
    mammary, 44
    prostate, 37, 38, 39, 40, 151
    sebaceous, 100
    sweat, 106, 129
Glucose, 83, 85, 86
Glyceryl guaiacolate, 60

Glycogen, 210
Gonorrhea, 211
Gout, 22
    symptoms, 22

H

Hair
    brushing, 99
    dry, 97-100
    oily, 174-175
    thinning, 160
Hay fever. *See* Allergies.
HDL cholesterol, 87, 136, 141
Headaches, 117-124
    cluster, 119
    diet in treatment of,
      122-123
    migraine, 117, 119
    relaxation exercises for, 120
Heart
    arrhythmia, 107
    attacks, 134-135
    failure, 143, 200
Heartburn, 124-128
    symptoms, 124, 126
Heat, and dry skin, 100-104
Heat treatment
    in arthritis, 26
    for back pain, 32
    in bladder infection, 39
    in breast pain, 46
    in headaches, 119
Heimlich maneuver, 125
Help for Incontinent People
    (HIP), 150
Hemorrhoids, 128-134
    external, 129
    internal, 128-129
    in pregnancy, 129
    prolapsed, 129
    treatment, 130-134
Herbal remedies, 56
Heredity
    and cholesterol, 135
    and dry skin, 100
    and hemorrhoids, 129
    and hypertension, 143
    in menstrual cramps, 167
    and varicose veins, 196
Hernia, hiatal, 126
High blood cholesterol, 134-143
High blood pressure, 143-150, 337

INDEX

INDEX

Teeth *(continued)*
    sensitive, 193
Tests
    cardiovascular screening, 89
    exercise, 89
Therapy
    estrogen replacement, 162
    hormone, 44, 162
    root-canal, 193
Thermometers, 108
Thirst
    in diabetes, 82, 83
    increased, 92
Throat,
    sore, 59, 60
    strep, 58
Thrombophlebitis, 200
Thyroid, underactive, 63
Toenails, trimming, 68
Toothache, 192-195
Transient ischemic attack (TIA),
    144
Traveler's diarrhea, 92, 96
Trichomonas, 211
Triglycerides, 136
Tumors, fibroid, 162
Tyramine, 122-123

U

Ulcers
    duodenal, 126
    stomach, 126
Ultraviolet light, 55
Urethral plugs, 153-154
Uterus, retroverted, 169

V

Vaginal
    discharge, 209-211

Vaginal *(continued)*
    dryness, 161, 163
    soreness, 163
Vaginitis, 83
Vaginosis, 211
Vaporizers, 59, 103
Varicose veins, 195-201
    pelvic, 167
Vaseline. *See* Petrolatum.
Viruses
    common cold, 56
    flu, 112
Vision
    blurred, 83
    changes in, 117
    loss of, 144
Vitamin A, 65, 70, 133
Vitamin B_6, 172
Vitamin C, 59, 198
Vitamin D, 65, 181
Vitamin E, 65
Vitamin K, 65
Vomiting, 172-174

W

Warts, perianal, 130
Weaning, 52
Weight
    in arthritis, 27
    in diabetes, 82, 83, 86
    gain, 201-209
    and hemorrhoids, 129, 134
    and hypertension, 145
    in incontinence, 153
    loss in diabetes, 83
    and varicose veins, 197

Y

Yeast infections, 209-215